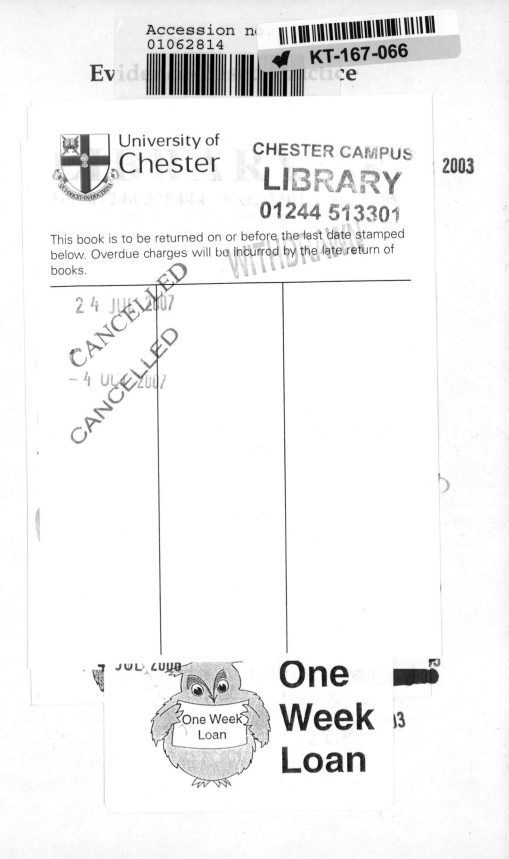

Evidence-Based Practice

A CRITICAL APPRAISAL

Edited by
Liz Trinder

with
Shirley Reynolds

b

**Blackwell
Science**

© 2000 Blackwell Science Ltd
Editorial Offices:
Osney Mead, Oxford OX2 0EL
25 John Street, London WC1N 2BL
23 Ainslie Place, Edinburgh EH3 6AJ
350 Main Street, Malden
  MA 02148 5018, USA
54 University Street, Carlton
  Victoria 3053, Australia
10 rue Casimir Delavigne
  75006 Paris, France

Other Editorial Offices:

Blackwell Wissenschafts-Verlag GmbH
Kurfürstendamm 57
10707 Berlin, Germany

Blackwell Science KK
MG Kodenmacho Building
7–10 Kodenmacho Nihombashi
Chuo-ku, Tokyo 104, Japan

The right of the Author to be identified as the
Author of this Work has been asserted in
accordance with the Copyright, Designs and
Patents Act 1988.

First published 2000

Set in 10 on 12.5pt Palatino
by DP Photosetting, Aylesbury, Bucks
Printed and bound in Great Britain at
The Alden Press, Oxford and Northampton

The Blackwell Science logo is a trade mark of
Blackwell Science Ltd, registered at the
United Kingdom Trade Marks Registry

DISTRIBUTORS

Marston Book Services Ltd
PO Box 269
Abingdon
Oxon OX14 4YN
(*Orders:* Tel: 01235 465500
      Fax: 01235 465555)

USA
Blackwell Science, Inc.
Commerce Place
350 Main Street
Malden, MA 02148 5018
(*Orders:* Tel: 800 759 6102
       781 388 8250
      Fax: 781 388 8255)

Canada
Login Brothers Book Company
324 Saulteaux Crescent
Winnipeg, Manitoba R3J 3T2
(*Orders:* Tel: 204 837-2987
      Fax: 204 837-3116)

Australia
Blackwell Science Pty Ltd
54 University Street
Carlton, Victoria 3053
(*Orders:* Tel: 03 9347 0300
      Fax: 03 9347 5001)

A catalogue record for this title is available
from the British Library

ISBN 0-632-05058-6

Library of Congress
Cataloging-in-Publication Data

Evidence-based practice: a critical appraisal/
edited by Liz Trinder with Shirley Reynolds.
    p.; cm.
    Includes bibliographical references and
index.
    ISBN 0-632-05058-6 (pbk.)
    1. Evidence-based medicine. 2. Primary
care (medicine) I. Trinder, Liz.
II. Reynolds, Shirley
    [DNLM: 1. Evidence-Based Medicine.
WB 102 E934 2000]
RA 427. E935 2000
362.1 – dc21

                              99-059641

For further information on Blackwell Science,
visit our website:
www.blackwell-science.com

Contents

List of Contributors

Richard Blomfield, RGN BA(Hons), MA   Lecturer in Nursing, School of Nursing and Midwifery, University of East Anglia

Rob B. Briner, BSc, MSc, PhD   Senior Lecturer in Organizational Psychology, Birkbeck College, University of London, London

John R. Geddes, MD, MRCPsych   Senior Clinical Research Fellow and Honorary Consultant Psychiatrist, Dept of Psychiatry, University of Oxford

J. A. Muir Grey, CBE, MD   Director, Institute of Health Sciences, University of Oxford

Martyn Hammersley, BSc, MA, PhD   Professor of Educational and Social Research, School of Education, The Open University, Milton Keynes

Sally E. Hardy, RGN, RMN, BA(Hons), MSc   Lecturer, Schools of Health (Nursing & Midwifery), University of East Anglia, Norwich

Toby Lipman, MBBS, MRCGP   General Practitioner and NHSE Northern and Yorkshire Research Training Fellow, Westerhope Medical Group, Newcastle-upon-Tyne

Shirley A. Reynolds, BSc, MSc, C Clin Psychol, PhD   Senior Lecturer in Clinical Psychology/Co-Director Doctoral Programme in Clinical Psychology, School of Health Policy and Practice, University of East Anglia, Norwich

Liz Trinder, BA, PhD   Lecturer in Social Work Research, School of Social Work, University of East Anglia, Norwich

Chapter 1

Introduction: the Context of Evidence-Based Practice

Liz Trinder

Introduction

The emergence of evidence-based practice has to be one of the success stories of the 1990s. In the space of ten years the movement has had a significant impact on health care and policy. In the UK there are centres, amongst others, for evidence-based medicine, evidence-based child services and mental health services. This organisational framework has been accompanied by a panoply of practice manuals, journals and newsletters, toolkits and software packages, websites and e-mail discussion groups. The depth of influence within UK medicine has been paralleled by a breadth of expansion internationally. The movement has rapidly become a global phenomenon transcending national boundaries. An international network to support the development of evidence-based medicine has developed swiftly in the form of the Cochrane Collaboration, which now has centres in the UK and continental Europe, North and South America, Africa, Asia and Australasia.

Although the emergence of evidence-based medicine has been rapid and dramatic, just as extraordinary has been the adoption of the key concepts of evidence-based medicine in other disciplines and professions under the generic title of evidence-based practice. Over the last few years evidence-based approaches have been developed in most health fields, including evidence-based dentistry, nursing, public health, physiotherapy and mental health. Progress has not stopped there: uniquely it would appear that an approach originating in medicine is being advocated and adopted in more distant fields of professional activity, including social work, probation, education and human resource management.

The purpose of this book is to stand back from the flurry of excitement and activity that has accompanied the development of evidence-based practice, and to take stock of what has occurred and what challenges remain for the diverse fields of professional activity that have engaged or are beginning to engage with evidence-based practice. The book aims to address three major questions:

(1) What is evidence-based practice?

The roots of evidence-based practice can be found in the emergence of evidence-based medicine in the early 1990s. Chapter 2 provides an introduction to the core concepts, processes and procedures of evidence-based medicine and should be a starting point for those who are unfamiliar with its basic principles. Over the last few years many other disciplines within and outside of medicine have adopted the 'evidence-based' tag and can therefore be considered under the generic title of 'evidence-based practice'. The book as a whole presents individual case studies to show how evidence-based practice is being developed within primary care, mental health, public health, nursing, social work and probation, education and human resource management. Each case study outlines what evidence-based practice initiatives are being developed within particular disciplines and how evidence-based practice is being defined or interpreted.

One of the strengths of the case-study approach is that it makes it possible to compare and contrast the varied stages of development, and varied interpretations, of the concept of evidence-based practice across the disciplines. What becomes apparent is that in the disciplines closest to hospital medicine (general practice, mental health, public health) the development of evidence-based practice both appears to most closely resemble the original formulation of evidence-based medicine, as well as to have progressed furthest. Elsewhere, the notion of evidence-based practice has been subject to considerable reinterpretation (most notably in social work and probation) and, despite the presence of some powerful advocates, has met with a higher degree of ambivalence or resistance. The appropriateness of this variation is considered in Chapter 10.

(2) What are the strengths and weaknesses of evidence-based practice?

Although the rise and expansion of evidence-based practice has been spectacular, it has been accompanied by considerable criticism from opponents, both in medicine and in other fields. Supporters and advocates of evidence-based practice claim that the approach results in the best practice and the best use of resources. In contrast, opponents have countered with claims that evidence-based practice is a covert method of rationing resources, is overly simplistic and constrains professional autonomy. In particular, critics have pointed out that there is no evidence that evidence-based practice actually works. Contributors were therefore asked, in the case studies chosen, to outline the responses to evidence-based practice in their discipline from practitioners, managers, researchers and consumers, as well as to provide their personal perspectives on the relevance and helpfulness of evidence-based practice. What is immediately apparent is that there is limited consensus on the merits of evidence-based practice. Chapter 10 outlines these divisions between the champions and critics of evidence-based practice and undertakes the difficult, and controversial task of critically appraising the strengths and weaknesses of evidence-based practice as a cross-disciplinary approach.

(3) How can we explain the emergence and spread of evidence-based practice?

It is unusual for ideas emerging from practitioner researchers to have such a dramatic and widespread impact on policy and practice, and it merits investigation. The individual case studies outline some of the background conditions that have presaged the adoption of evidence-based practice. The remainder of this chapter draws these threads together and looks more broadly at the similar background conditions that have prompted and facilitated the widespread endorsement of evidence-based practice. The core argument is that the emergence and rapid expansion of evidence-based practice must be understood against a background of increasing preoccupation with managing risk, critiques of science and professionalism and the emergence of managerialism and consumerism.

Why has evidence-based practice emerged?

It might seem rather an odd task to try to examine the reasons for the emergence of evidence-based practice. Certainly for those within the movement, and for many of those outside, its very success seems to be a clear indication that it is quite simply a self-evidently good idea. Evidence-based practice relays a devastatingly effective and simple message: the argument that practice should be based on the most up-to-date, valid and reliable research findings has an instant intuitive appeal, and is so obviously sensible and rational that it is difficult to resist.

Enthusiasts of evidence-based practice argue remarkably clearly and consistently across the disciplines, with four main points emerging:

(1) Research–practice gap

A common refrain in all the case study chapters, and in wider evidence-based practice and in professional literature, is the limited extent to which professionals utilise or draw upon research findings to determine or guide their actions. Instead it is suggested that professionals rely upon a range of other, less reliable, indicators such as:

- knowledge gained during primary training
- prejudice and opinion

- outcomes of previous cases
- fads and fashions
- advice of senior and not so senior colleagues.

(2) *Poor quality of much research*

In addition, it is argued that much of the research that is available is methodologically weak, in particular that it is not based on the 'gold standard' of well-conducted randomised controlled trial (RCT) designs, or is inapplicable within clinical or practice situations. This argument is made by exponents of evidence-based medicine, as well as within other areas of professional practice including social work, probation, education and human resource management.

(3) *Information overload*

The sheer quantity of research available, however, creates problems in itself. Particularly in medicine, practitioners are unable to keep up with the continuing global output of research findings, nor do they have the skills or means to be able to distinguish between rigorous and useful research, and poor or unreliable research.

(4) *Practice which is not evidence-based*

The consequence of factors (1) to (3) is that practitioners continue to utilise interventions which have been shown to be ineffective or harmful, that there is a slow or limited adoption of interventions which have been proven to be effective or more effective, and that there continue to be variations in practice.

Allied to the clarity and intuitive appeal is the portability factor. Evidence-based practice has its origins in medicine but is essentially a process or methodology, and one which claims a neutral, almost context-less stance. Hence the process appears capable of expansion to a wide range of disciplines involving human services, and even beyond (e.g. evidence-based veterinary practice or evidence-based agriculture). Given the research–practice gap reported in many disciplines, the low utilisation of research by practitioners and criticisms of the relevance of academic research, the evidence-based practice approach appears to have offered a tailor-made solution to these problems, and one which has been readily adopted throughout the health professions and beyond.

Although the obvious merits of a practice based clearly on good evidence and the tireless work of advocates can explain some of the success of evidence-based practice, these factors alone cannot provide a sufficient explanation. Other good ideas have not succeeded in the same way, nor have other equally dedicated groups of professionals been so influential so quickly. Instead, this section will examine a range of other factors. In essence, the argument is that evidence-based practice has developed so quickly because both its central concerns and the form that it takes resonates with and mirrors significant contemporary issues and concerns, namely those of risk, audit and effectiveness, rationalism, transparency, professional accountability, consumerism, empowerment and the needs of the information society. Evidence-based practice is quite simply a product of its time. The following sections therefore examine the context within which evidence-based practice has developed, examining two distinct, though related trends – the emergence of the risk society and the 'appliance of science'; and the emergence of managerialism and the audit society.

The risk society

A current preoccupation of social theory is the extent to which we are living in changing times. Debate will continue as to whether we are living in high modern or post-modern times, nonetheless most commentators would concur that contemporary society is characterised by dramatic social change, occurring at an ever increasing pace. Further, this degree of change is associated with a heightened awareness of risk and a preoccupation with its management (Beck 1992), culminating in an 'age of anxiety' (Dunnant & Porter 1996). Science, and public perceptions of science, play a crucial role in this.

The work of Anthony Giddens (1991, 1993, 1994), one of the foremost contemporary social theorists, is highly pertinent to understanding the development of evidence-based practice. Giddens argues that in traditional societies a sense of 'ontological security' (the confidence people have in their self-identity and social and material environments) was anchored firmly in the locality, in the kinship system, the local community, religion and tradition. Now in contrast, Giddens argues that we are living in a time of endings and transitions, with the emergence of a post-traditional society. Instead of fixed and locally based traditions, post-traditional societies are subject to and shaped by globalised, rather than local, social and economic forces. The traditional authorities of the past, in particular the church, are far less influential, and social bonds are increasingly made by individuals in particular situations (reflecting 'lifestyle choices'), rather than inherited from the past. The changes in family forms, the rise in divorce and single-parenting and the declining role of the extended family are just some illustrations of this.

Perhaps the most important consequence of the shift to post-traditional societies for our discussion of evidence-based practice is the notion of risk. In pre-modern times Giddens points to the centrality of concepts of 'fortuna' (fortune or fate) where catastrophe was attributed to acts of god or nature. In post-traditional times there is a heightened sense of risk, coupled with a sense that contingencies are generally humanly created, as well as inescapable. The transformation of human activity in modern times requires considerable and constant amounts of trust in expert systems (what Giddens terms 'abstract systems') (Giddens 1991). Even the relatively simple task of driving to work requires the lay person to trust numerous unknown others, including other drivers, as well as car manufacturers and repairers, traffic planners and driving test examiners. It is impossible for either individuals or organisations to avoid externally generated risks, ranging from food additives and genetically modified food to stock market crashes and political upheaval. The results are unsettling.

The promise of modernity, however, is that risk can be assessed and controlled by expert knowledge, or at least procedures put in place to minimise risks (Giddens 1994: 111). Yet although we are ever more dependent upon science, we appear increasingly aware of its limitations. Our confidence in science and experts is tempered by two factors. First, there is a recognition that many risks are generated by the very expert systems which we are required to trust. Second, given the very fluidity of modern life, and the constant re-examination of tradition and social practices, there are no guarantees that particular bits of knowledge will not be revised (Giddens 1991: 39–40). Giddens argues that although lay people are required to trust experts this trust is typically ambivalent, a bargain with modernity 'governed by specific admixtures of deference and scepticism, comfort and fear' and founded upon a recognition of the limitations of expertise (Giddens 1994: 90).

One particular and pertinent example is the critique of professionalism over the last two decades. Whilst it would be easy to overstate the degree of this critique, it is certainly the case that the esteem in which professionals, including doctors, were held in the earlier part of the twentieth century has diminished – though ironically standards of practice would be generally higher now than in previous decades. Criticisms of professional competence, discretion and self-regulation have come from policy-makers and managers (see under *Managerialism and the audit society* below). From lay sources, the growth of consumer and self-help groups, coupled with intensive media scrutiny, have led to charges of paternalism as well as a challenge to claims of a monopoly of expertise. More recently internal critiques have also emerged, including the pessimistic 'nothing works' found in probation (see Chapter 7), as well as the growth of the evidence-based practice movement.

The 'appliance of science'

If Anthony Giddens and many other commentators are correct when they identify a crisis of belief in science and expertise, why has a movement so

firmly based in science and rationality been so successful? This is particularly interesting at a time when the *social* sciences have moved in
precisely the opposite direction, away from the positivism of the post-war
years, to emphasise the socially constructed and therefore fluid and
uncertain nature of knowledge (e.g. see Lyotard 1984). Some of these
concerns have been echoed in medicine (e.g. see Marinker 1996; Greenhalgh & Hurwitz 1998) although their influence is limited compared to the
momentum of the evidence-based practice movement. Elsewhere, in social
work, education and medicine, the influence of the social sciences is more
substantial and can partly account for the much more muted acceptance of
evidence-based practice (see Chapters 6, 7 and 8).

Again Giddens is helpful in providing an explanation for the emergence
of a scientific movement. He argues that four adaptive reactions are possible when questioning traditional authorities and expert systems (1991:
135–7):

- *Pragmatic acceptance*: where there is an assumption that risks cannot be
  controlled and so temporary solutions are sought amidst underlying
  anxiety
- *Cynical pessimism*: a world-weary or humorous response to risk, and
  celebration of the here-and-now
- *Radical engagement*: where action rather than rational analysis and discussion are used to challenge perceived sources of danger – e.g. the
  environmental movement
- *Sustained optimism*: a position of faith.

It is the fourth strategy, of sustained optimism, that is most relevant to the
discussion of evidence-based practice. Giddens defines sustained optimism as a position where continued faith is held in reason and science, and,
despite public ambivalence, there is a belief that experts can find social and
technological solutions for major problems and that rational thought, and
especially science, still offers the best sources of long-term security.

The development of evidence-based practice fits squarely within Giddens' strategy of sustained optimism. Evidence-based practice has
emerged within a context where there is a heightened sense of risk, and
increasingly reliance upon as well as increased distrust of expertise.
However, rather than rejecting or questioning science, evidence-based
practice requires that a much more rigorous science should be applied far
more systematically by practitioners. In a context where the competence of
practitioners is being questioned more than ever – witness the furore over
the Bristol pediatric heart surgeons – the solution is to turn to science more,
rather than less. Evidence-based practice remains firmly committed
therefore to the modernist promise that risk can be assessed and controlled
by expert knowledge, meaning in this context that the potential harm of

interventions is minimised and the potential benefits maximised. This requires more rather than less science, and new mechanisms for risk management.

The question is what sort of science does this require? In a risk-conscious world tinged with doubt and scepticism about science and expertise, Beck (1992) argues that the goal of science has shifted from a positive goal of social change to a defensive attempt to protect from harm where risk assessment becomes central, but by its very nature imperfect. According to Beck, there has been a shift from a confident 'primary scientisation' or science of discovery, to a more cautious 'reflexive scientisation' based on an incremental model which resists challenge. What evidence-based practice does is to provide a methodology and set of procedures to produce an incrementally developing, but endlessly revisable, body of knowledge, rather than big theories or authoritative figures.

Managerialism and the audit society

The second major influence on the emergence of evidence-based practice has been the significant changes that have occurred in public services in many western democracies in the last two decades. The cluster of developments which have occurred, including the rise of managerialism, the emphasis on value-for-money and the growth of audit have all contributed to shaping the goals and form of evidence-based practice.

Alongside the preoccupation with risk, the last two decades have also witnessed the emergence of audit and managerialism in many western democracies. Since the mid-1970s, significant changes in the organisation, practice and culture of public services have occurred. From the late 1970s the impetus for change was initially driven by requirements to rein in the burgeoning growth in public expenditure. Yet the changes have now moved far beyond attempts to exert tighter fiscal control. Instead we have also witnessed the emergence of neo-liberal ideologies of micro-government, political discourses of accountability and performance, and economic discourses of value-for-money, including economy, efficiency and effectiveness (Power 1997: 43–4). In effect, what has occurred is a significant shift towards giving managers the right to manage, instituting systems of regulation to achieve value-for-money (economy, efficiency and effectiveness), and thereby producing accountability to the taxpayer and customer. In contrast to the period of expansion and growth in the 1950s and 1960s, the issue of value-for-money, including effectiveness, has become a central goal for public services (see Chapter 5). Thus over the last 20 years, a whole raft of reforms have been introduced in public services, framed within a managerialist discourse of responsibility, transparency, efficiency and customer orientation and accompanied by charters, missions, visions and performance tables (Clarke & Newman 1997: 35).

This shift towards managerialism is based on an explicit critique of the three traditional authorities of the post-war welfare state – the triumvirate of political representatives, bureaucrats and professionals. Where resources are finite and demands potentially endless and conflicting, managerialism has been presented as the solution which can rise above politics, of interfering politicians or self-interested professionals, in the interests of rational, efficient and accountable decision-making about resources (Clarke *et al.* 1994; Clarke & Newman 1997).

The real impact of managerialism, however, has been on the *processes* for target-setting, regulation and monitoring introduced throughout the public services in support of value-for-money objectives. The introduction of the medical audit and the Citizens Charter are just two examples. Not only are these developments important in terms of their objective of achieving value-for-money, they are also important in the sense that the achievement of value-for-money is sought through the introduction of processes, which in turn are presented as rational, non-political, neutral and transparent (Power 1997).

Michael Power's (1997) analysis of the rise of what he terms the 'audit society' is helpful in identifying why such a major shift towards issues of effectiveness, accountability and transparency has occurred. Mirroring Giddens' analysis, Power argues that the explosion of auditable management control systems has occurred at a time when there is a heightened awareness of risk and a diminution of trust in experts. The solution has been to lessen reliance upon experts and instead to transfer trust into audit systems. An apparently greater sense of safety and control is thus generated as the emphasis shifts, from trust in individuals, towards an audit of the quality of expert services.

Similar concerns and processes are observable with evidence-based practice. Power, in a definition that might equally apply to evidence-based practice, notes that:

> 'The audit explosion is to do with the need to install a publicly auditable self-inspecting capacity with attempts to link ideals of accountability to those of self-learning'.
>
> (Power 1997: 67)

The focus on effectiveness, though to a far lesser degree efficiency and economy, is the central driving force of evidence-based practice. It is also clear that the focus on proceduralisation and the types of procedures involved in evidence-based practice mirrors many of the managerial reforms introduced over the last two decades. As we argued above, the core of evidence-based practice is its procedures rather than its substantive output. In its few short years, the Cochrane Collaboration, for example, has generated an astounding array of procedures, checklists and guidelines spanning the entire process from identifying evidence (including procedures for hand-searching), through evaluating evidence, collating and summarising evidence, to presenting and updating reviews of evidence. Like audit systems, the main rationale behind proceduralisation provided by the Cochrane Collaboration and other evidence-based practice initiatives, is a requirement to make every attempt to exclude bias and to ensure accountability and transparency, through the institution of standardised, rational and neutral procedures.

Giddens (1993) argues that in an uncertain world, social institutions ward off externally generated disturbances by becoming increasingly self-referential and inward-looking through what he terms the 'sequestration of experience'. The reaction to the messiness and uncertainty of individual patients/clients and situations is to establish boundaries outside which alternative ideas and experiences are set. In the case of evidence-based practice, alternative methodologies and ideas are excluded by procedure. The potential messiness of the real world – patients with multiple and complex conditions – is met by a battery of procedures designed to render the complex manageable through the procedural production of evidence. Challenges to the approach are met by further proceduralisation utilising the same rationale. Thus, for example, a system is being set up to prevent and manage conflicts which occur within the Cochrane Collaboration by the creation of a conflict support group, an internal ombudsman, and a document on handling and resolving conflict (Cochrane Collaboration 1998b).

Professionalism, empowerment and consumerism

Our argument so far has been that evidence-based practice has emerged in the context of significant change in public services, prompted by the concern with effectiveness and proceduralisation combined with a critique of professional expertise. We have also highlighted the similarities between the goals and processes of evidence-based practice and managerial changes within public services. We are then left with a puzzle as to why evidence-based practice began as a professional activity. If recent changes in public services have had placing greater control over professional discretion as one of their primary goals, why are evidence-based practitioners adopting methods that mirror – in their processes and rationality – managerial interventions? Indeed one of the constituencies where evidence-based practice has had most success is with health service managers, who have provided considerable support and funding for evidence-based practice initiatives, as well as endorsement and utilisation of evidence-based practice outputs (Grahame-Smith 1995).

Part of the explanation for the overlap between the managerial and evidence-based practice agenda is that changes in public services have focused on ensuring that concern with performance and effectiveness is dispersed throughout organisations and not confined to management as strictly defined (Clarke *et al.* 1994; Clarke & Newman 1997; Power 1997). The mechanisms by which this has occurred have included recruiting professionals into management positions, devolving management systems (e.g. GP fundholding) and the introduction of audit and performance mechanisms. Thus Clarke & Newman (1997: 35) can declare 'we are all managers now'.

It would be a mistake, however, to regard evidence-based practice merely as a managerial Trojan horse. Clarke & Newman's (1997: 31) analysis of the process of managerial dispersal suggests that the aim of managerialism is to break up traditional areas of power, including professional power, but they add that the process of dispersal also inevitably produces new sites of resistance. One of the major battlegrounds has indeed been over quality. Clarke and Newman argue that the influence of professionalism has not been completely displaced. Instead there has been contestation, where managers using a quality agenda seek to subsume professional autonomy for organisational efficiency, whilst, at the same time, professionals use a quality agenda to defend professional values and user interests (1997: 81, 119). They identify two means whereby this occurs (1997: 76):

- *Subordination*: where professional judgement has to be framed within the context of management of financial realities and responsibilities
- *Cooption*: managerial attempts to colonise the terrain of professional discourse, by, for example, incorporating service quality issues into corporate missions and strategies.

With evidence-based practice, however, we can recognise a third, and initially professional-led, strategy. Both Clarke & Newman (1997: 119) and Power (1997: 50–51) argue that so far, managerialism has focused on issues of economy and efficiency, with relatively less attention to quality and effectiveness. Evidence-based practice has rapidly developed in this gap to produce a professional-defined and led strategy that promises effectiveness. Thus evidence-based practice can be viewed as a radical strategy where professionals fight back and challenge managerial definitions of effectiveness.

Its radicalism takes other forms too. As well as the challenge to managerialism, it also throws down the gauntlet to other traditional authorities, the leaders of professions steeped in experience and authority but not necessarily in the best evidence. In the emphasis on self-learning, and the belief that anyone can learn the skills of evidence-based practice, it is potentially therefore a radically democratising strategy where the most junior members of the profession can be as skilled in identifying the evidence as the most respected. Evidence rather than experience becomes priviliged.

Evidence-based practice is not just framed as a means to empower individual professionals but also as a mechanism to deliver the safest and most effective interventions for customers and enhance customer choice. Attention to the consumer is of course another of the key watchwords of the late twentieth century, particularly in the neo-liberal form of the consumer as a rational agent exercising freedom, choice and personal responsibility. The emphasis on the customer is evident in a number of ways. First, evidence-based practice promises greater accountability to the consumer by the provision of best evidence. Second, the Cochrane Collaboration has worked hard to involve consumers and consumer groups, through its consumer network and through attempts to provide accessible summaries of evidence. The reformulation of evidence-based practice to incorporate attention to patient wishes within clinical decision-making, alongside evidence and clinical experience (Sackett *et al.* 1996) might prove more problematic.

The information society

In seeking to question why evidence-based practice has emerged at this moment in time, it is worth looking briefly at technological change and the information society. The explosion of medical information, and the inability of practitioners to digest it, is frequently given as one of the reasons for the development of evidence-based practice (Sackett & Haynes 1995; Haines & Haines 1998). The movement has turned this to its advantage; indeed evidence-based practice would not be possible without the developments in information technology, especially electronic databases and the Internet, which have enabled its practitioners to identify, collate, disseminate and access evidence on a global scale. It has also facilitated the establishment and maintenance of an international organisation like the Cochrane Collaboration, with Cochrane centres and review groups scattered across the globe but united by the Internet and a standardised procedure.

A product of its time

The timing of evidence-based practice is therefore not accidental. It has developed within a specific context, particularly the current preoccupations with risk, ambivalence about science and professional expertise, and the concern with effectiveness, proceduralisation and the consumer. Much of the initial success of evidence-based practice can be attributed to its ability to both endorse and redefine some of these concerns, drawing them all together within a coherent and tightly bound package.

The response to the critique of science is to place renewed emphasis on science with a constantly revisable and transparent process that excludes uncertainty and, in an age of anxiety, promises security for practitioners, researchers, managers and consumers. Trust is transferred from the fallible individual and placed in the revised system. In response to the emergence of managerialism, the explosion of audit systems and challenges to professionalism, evidence-based practice has offered a professional solution, itself based upon an even more transparent, neutral and rational process, and one which also claims to represent the interests of, and involve, the customer or consumer. The ability to pull together potentially contradictory but dominant concerns into a seamless self-referential package, fully utilising advances in information technology, has made evidence-based practice difficult to challenge.

Nor is the original location or host for evidence-based practice an accident. It is unlikely that evidence-based practice could have emerged anywhere other than medicine. Two factors contribute to this: nowhere else is there a profession so historically powerful, nor with such a strong scientific research tradition, both of which have been crucial to the content and development of evidence-based practice.

The expansion of evidence-based practice

As is clear from the contributions to this book the pattern of influence and uptake of evidence-based practice has not, however, been uniform. Acute medicine is in effect the epicentre of the movement towards evidence-based practice. Those disciplines closest to this epicentre – other medical specialisms, primary care, mental health – are those which have adopted evidence-based practice most enthusiastically, and with least redefinition. Within the health professions, one of the factors which has facilitated the rapid expansion of evidence-based practice has been the issue of proximity. Evidence-based practice has had its most receptive audience when that audience is one where there are considerable educational, occupational and organisational overlaps with the originating discipline or specialism. Access to the concepts and processes of evidence-based practice has been facilitated by people working in the same organisations, reading some of the same journals and having access to the same training events. In the UK this has been given further impetus by NHS initiatives such as the Centre for Reviews and Dissemination at the University of York. As well as physical proximity, the swift endorsement of evidence-based practice has also been based on cultural proximity, referencing a common language and research tradition.

Neither of these factors – physical and cultural proximity – is clearly present in disciplines such as human resource management, social work and education which occupy the outer edges. Furthest away from the medical epicentre the energy created begins to dissipate and the impact is more muted and less consistent. Indeed, the further from the centre – in education, social work and human resource management – the more limited the degree of commitment to evidence-based practice and the higher degree of ambivalence, scepticism or even resistance. In the outer-edge disciplines the evidence-based practice message has resonated with small, relatively isolated groups who have been long advocating the adoption of a 'scientific' approach to practice – for example the empirical practitioners in social work and the school-effectiveness lobby in education. In each of these disciplines, however, the groups identifying with evidence-based practice fall largely outside the research mainstream of their disciplines, or are far less central or influential than in medicine. Instead these outer-edge professions have alternative, more influential research and practice traditions, with the result that positions taken on evidence-based practice reflect pre-existing ongoing arguments or research traditions within the discipline. Education, social work, human resource management and to some extent, nursing, each have fairly long-developed research traditions which clash with the central ontological, epistemological and methodological tenets of evidence-based practice. The methodological centre of gravity of these disciplines falls largely within the social sciences and qualitative or non-experimental quantitative research, in contrast to medical research where the balance is tilted strongly towards models of research practice and cumulativeness drawn from the natural sciences.

The following chapter by Shirley Reynolds outlines the core principles of evidence-based medicine and can be seen as establishing a baseline definition against which the development of evidence-based practice in other disciplines can be compared. In Chapter 3 Toby Lipman examines the development of evidence-based practice in primary care, emphasising the opportunities evidence-based practice gives for continuing self-directed learning of practitioners. John Geddes' contribution describes the development of evidence-based practice in the multidisciplinary arena of mental health, illustrating both the opportunities for improved practice as well as some of the difficulties in an area where the performance of different professional groups is being compared head to head. In Chapter 5 Muir Gray, one of the leading figures in the development of evidence-based health care, tracks the emergence of evidence-based health care and argues strongly for the importance of making health care decisions which are based on the best available evidence. The following chapters reveal a greater degree of ambivalence about evidence-based practice. In Chapter 6 Richard Blomfield and Sally Hardy note the long history of the subservience of nursing as a profession and express concern that the importation of a scientific model will inhibit the work done by nursing on reflective practice or do justice to the caring aspects of nursing.

In Chapter 7 I look at the emergence of evidence-based practice in probation and social work. In social work the concept has received a mixed response, with enthusiastic adherents drawing on earlier traditions of empirical practice as well as a rather tongue-in-cheek adoption of the name but not the methodological content of evidence-based practice by the more influential group of pragmatist researchers. In probation, by contrast, a narrow managerially led push towards evidence-based practice is being advanced rapidly. In Chapter 8, Martyn Hammersley offers a critique of the early calls for the development of evidence-based education, and in particular questions the relevance of the model for education where practice is primarily based on practical rather than technical decisions.

The last case study, on human resource management by Rob Briner, is the only area of practice that falls substantially outside the public sector and is also the area where evidence-based practice is least developed. He identifies the poor quality of much research in the area of human resource management and argues for, but recognises the barriers to, the development of evidence-based human resource management. The final chapter, Chapter 10, attempts to appraise evidence-based practice critically as a generic cross-disciplinary phenomenon. It examines some of the practical and conceptual difficulties with evidence-based practice and identifies some of the challenges that evidence-based practice has yet to resolve if it is to meet its goal of raising the quality of research and practice.

References

Beck U. (1992) *Risk Society: Towards a New Modernity*. Sage, London.

Carr-Hill R. (1995) Welcome? to the brave new world of evidence-based medicine. *Social Science and Medicine*, **41**, 1467–8.

Charlton B. (1995) Megatrials are subordinate to medical science. *British Medical Journal*, **311**, 257.

Clarke J., Cochrane A. & McLaughlin E. (1994) The impact of managerialization. In J. Clarke, A. Cochrane & E. McLaughlin (eds) *Managing Social Policy*. Sage, London.

Cochrane Collaboration (1998a) *Cochrane Collaboration Prompts Changes*. Url: http://hiru.mcmaster.ca/cochrane/cochrane/ccimpact.htm.

Cochrane Collaboration (1998b) *Steering Group Minutes*. Baltimore, 20th, 22nd and 25th October 1998. URL: http://hiru.mcmaster.ca/cochrane/cochrane/201098.htm.

Court C. (1996) NHS Handbook criticises evidence-based medicine. *British Medical Journal*, **312**, 1439–40.

Dunnant S. & Porter R. (1996) *The Age of Anxiety*. Virago, London.

Gabe J., Kelleher D. & Williams G. (1994) *Challenging Medicine*. Routledge, London.

Giddens A. (1991) *The Consequences of Modernity*. Polity, Cambridge.

Giddens A. (1993) *Modernity and Self-Identity*. Polity, Cambridge.

Giddens A. (1994) Living in a Post-Traditional Society. In U. Beck, A. Giddens & S. Lash (eds) *Reflexive Modernisation*. Polity, Cambridge.

Grahame-Smith D. (1995) Evidence-based medicine: Socratic dissent. *British Medical Journal*, **310**, 1126–7.

Greenhalgh T. & Hurwitz, B. (1998) *Narrative-Based Medicine: Dialogue and Discourse in Clinical Practice*. BMJ Publishing Group, London.

Haines B. & Haines A. (1998) Barriers and bridges to evidence-based clinical practice. *British Medical Journal*, **317**, 273–6.

Jones G. & Sagar S. (1995) No guidance is provided for situations for which evidence is lacking. *British Medical Journal*, **311**, 258.

Lancet (1995) Evidence-based medicine, in its place [Editorial]. *Lancet*, **346**, 785.

Lyotard J. (1984) *The Postmodern Condition: A Report on Knowledge*. Manchester University Press, Manchester.

Marinker M. (ed.) *Sense and Sensibility in Health Care*. BMJ Publishing Group, London.

Power M. (1997) *The Audit Society: Rituals of Verification*. Oxford University Press, Oxford.

Sackett D. & Haynes R. (1995) On the need for evidence-based medicine. *Evidence-Based Medicine*, **1**, 5.

Sackett D.L., Rosenberg W.M.C., Gray J.A.M., Haynes R.B. & Richardson W.S. (1996) Evidence-based medicine: what it is and what it isn't. *British Medical Journal*, **312**, 71–2.

Shahar, E. (1997) A Popperian perspective on the term 'evidence-based medicine'. *Journal of Evaluation in Clinical Practice*, **3**, 109–16.

Smith B. & Taylor R. (1996) Medicine: a healing or a dying art? *British Journal of General Practice*, **46**, 249–51.

Tannenbaum S. (1993) What physicians know. *New England Journal of Medicine*, **329**, 1268–71.

Taubes G. (1996) Looking for the evidence in medicine. *Science*, **272**, 22–4.

Chapter 2

The Anatomy of Evidence-Based Practice: Principles and Methods

Shirley Reynolds

Introduction

The impact of evidence-based medicine (EBM) on national policy in the UK has been remarkable. In less than a decade it has had a significant impact in many different professional groups and has become a cornerstone of UK health policy. The impact of evidence-based medicine has, to differing degrees, changed professional practice, influenced research activity and challenged professional identities in professions as diverse as medicine, social work, clinical psychology, nursing and education. The application of evidence-based medicine principles beyond medicine has resulted in the broadening of the core concept and the development of evidence-based practice (EBP), a title more suited to the interdisciplinary application of evidence-based medicine principles.

As the broader concept of evidence-based practice has emerged from the more focused concept of evidence-based medicine, so some of the initial principles may have been distorted or lost in the process. Inevitably, as dissemination occurs, different professional groups will interpret and adapt the concept of evidence-based medicine. This has the potential for considerable confusion. For this reason the aim of this chapter is to provide a brief overview only of the core features, principles and concepts of evidence-based medicine. There are many other more detailed sources of information about evidence-based medicine (e.g. Sackett *et al.* 1997, Grayson 1997); those requiring more detailed, specific information about evidence-based medicine may find the resouces listed in Box 2.1 useful. The first section of this chapter introduces the concept of evidence-based medicine and describes the background to the development of evidence-based medicine. The second section outlines the main procedures and methods used in evidence-based medicine. Some common concerns and problems with the concept of evidence-based medicine are highlighted in section three. Although evidence-based medicine has changed the culture of health service provision very markedly, these concerns may constrain

Box 2.1: Selected sources of information about evidence-based practice

Websites

The Cochrane Collaboration http://hiru.mcmaster.ca/COCHRANE/
OxamWeb http://www.psychiatry.ox.ac.uk/oxamweb/frames.html
ScHARR http://www.shef.ac.uk/uni/academic/R-Z/scharr/ir/netting.html
ACP Journal Club http://www.acponline.org/journals/acpjc/jcmenu.htm
NHS Centre for Reviews and Dissemination http://www.york.ac.uk/inst/crd/welcome.htm
UK Cochrane Centre http://www.cochrane.co.uk/

Discipline-specific websites

Centre for Evidence-Based Child Health http://www.ich.bpmf.ac.uk/ebm/ebm.htm
Centre for Evidence-Based Dentistry http://www.bhaoral.demon.co.uk/
Centre for Evidence-Based Nursing http://www.york.ac.uk/depts/hstd/centres/evidence/ev-intro.htm
Centre for Evidence-Based Medicine http://cebm.jr2.ox.ac.uk/
Centre for Evidence-Based Mental Health http://www.psychiatry.ox.ac.uk/cebmh/journal/
Centre for Evidence-Based Pharmacotherapy http://www.nottingham.ac.uk/~paxjc/clinphar.htm

Journals

Evidence-Based Medicine
Evidence-Based Mental Health
Evidence-Based Public Health
Evidence-Based Nursing
Bandolier
Clinical Evidence

CD-ROMs

Best Evidence
Cochrane Collaboration Library, Update Software, Oxford

the extent to which evidence-based medicine is effective in changing behaviours (see Box 2.1).

What is evidence-based practice?

The relationship between research and practice tends to be uneasy. Many professions claim to be based on knowledge derived from scientific endeavour. Despite this link, however, the translation of research findings to practice has frequently been erratic and unsystematic. This gap between research and practice can be quite literally life-threatening. For example, within medicine, Antman *et al.* (1992) demonstrated that the majority of contemporary medical textbooks recommended treatments for myocardial infarction which were of proven worthlessness, and that more recently developed treatments, of proven efficacy, were not recommended.

There are many possible reasons for this gap between research and practice. For example, doctors claim that research is frequently unrelated to their clinical concerns, that research does not help with the process of clinical decision-making, that research is inaccessible and difficult to understand, and that there is insufficient time in clinical practice to keep up to date with developments in clinical research. Similar concerns have been expressed amongst other professional groups, including clinical psychologists, nurses and social workers, as is evident from the chapters in this volume. The practical effect of this gap between research and professional practice is that dangerous or useless procedures continue to be implemented, and that effective, safe procedures are often introduced slowly into clinical practice, if at all. Furthermore, without an effective link between research and practice it is possible that research activities may become disengaged from the practical needs of clinical work and thus further fuel accusations that research does not help clinicians.

Supporters of evidence-based medicine claim that it has developed in order to bridge the gap between research and practice in medicine. Sackett *et al.* defined evidence-based medicine as:

> 'the conscientious, explicit and judicious use of current best evidence in making decisions about the care of individual patients, based on skills which allow the doctor to evaluate both personal experience and external evidence in a systematic and objective manner'.
>
> (Sackett *et al.* 1997: 71)

An important feature of evidence-based medicine is that in addition to providing an explicit statement of intent (what should happen), it goes further in providing a range of practical methods for overcoming the gap between research and clinical practice. First, evidence-based medicine distinguishes between research that is of direct clinical significance and that which is not. If research findings do not have an immediate practical relevance to clinicians they are marginal to the process of evidence-based medicine. This degree of clinical focus helps doctors to ignore the vast quantities of clinical research which are not of direct relevance to practice. Second, evidence-based medicine provides a set of simple rules for evaluating research evidence. These highly structured rules of critical appraisal provide a means by which non-researchers can engage with and challenge the complex presentation of clinical research reports. Third, evidence-based medicine provides a framework for making clinical decisions on the basis of research findings and of applying research findings to individual patients.

Evidence-based medicine provides all these advantages because it has harnessed the powerful tool of information technology. In this context the power of information technology lies in the fact that research evidence can be disseminated beyond hospital and university libraries directly to clinicians at their desks or in their clinics. Electronic communication makes it possible to link up with libraries, journals and research institutions via the Internet. Literature searches can now be performed without leaving the clinic, and selected information about high-quality research can now be directly accessed on CD-ROM and on the world-wide web (see above Box 2.1).

The concept of evidence-based medicine has a number of important components. First, it emphasises the professional responsibility of the doctor to use their judgement, personal experience, and also external evidence in making clinical decisions. Second, it refers explicitly to the care of *individual* patients, emphasising the primacy of the relationship between doctor and each individual (i.e. over that of the patient's family, the local community, the organisation in which health care is being provided, etc.) Third, it proposes that decision-making in clinical practice should be made explicit and thus be open to question and examination. Fourth, in stating that one should use 'the current best evidence' the definition of evidence-based medicine clearly suggests that evidence is always incomplete and subject to revision, that there are different types of evidence, and that there is a hierarchy of evidence (best to worst). Fifth, the definition refers to the need for systematic and objective evaluation, placing the clinician in a reflective and active role in relation to the patient, to the decision that is made, and to the doctor's own skills and judgement.

Background to the development of evidence-based medicine

The core features of evidence-based medicine, described above, reflect an ideological stance which is, to some extent, at odds with the hierarchical, status-driven stereotypes associated with medical practice. The core figure associated with the development of evidence-based medicine as a distinct movement was Archie Cochrane, who argued that since health care resources will always be limited, those resources should be used to provide health care services which have been shown to be effective (Cochrane 1972). Cochrane's contribution, however, went beyond simple considerations of rationalising the allocation of scarce resources. He wrote clearly, and from personal experience, about the primacy of the relationship between patient and doctor, the problems of applying research principles to health care, and the difficulties of applying the results of research trials to the care of individual patients (Cochrane 1972). Thus Cochrane combined a clinically oriented concern for the psychological and physical well-being of his patients, with a critical, research-orientated search for effective care.

Cochrane observed that although medicine had developed on the basis of advances in pure science, the application of scientific principles was largely absent in the evaluation of new treatment methods. Cochrane was one of the first in medicine to promote the use of randomised controlled trials (RCTs) in the evaluation of treatment methods and he pioneered the use of systematic reviews and meta-analyses in medicine. His influence in the UK National Health Service was profound: since Cochrane's death in 1988, the NHS has adopted his principles of systematic review and meta-analysis, and also contributed in 1992 to setting up the Cochrane Collaboration, an international initiative concerned with the preparation and dissemination of systematic reviews of health care research (Box 2.1).

A second important influence in evidence-based medicine were the developments in medical education at McMaster University in Canada. Medical education at McMaster was established in the 1960s, and pioneered teaching methods based on problem-based, self-directed learning (see Chapter 4). Central to this educational development was the integration of clinical practice with research, and the use of research principles to inform decisions about diagnosis, treatment and its side-effects, and prognosis. This new area of education was termed 'clinical epidemiology' (Sackett *et al.* 1991). Clinical epidemiology differed from traditional research teaching in that it was aimed not at *conducting* research, but at *using* research, i.e. applying research findings to clinical problems. Sackett and his colleagues argued that as scientific literature expands it becomes progressively more difficult for doctors to keep abreast of new methods of treatment or diagnosis. Thus, for example, Ramsey *et al.* (1991) demonstrated that there was a significant negative correlation between doctors' knowledge of up-to-date care, and the number of years that had elapsed since their graduation from medical school. Once doctors qualify, and after a period in practice, they tend to rely more on anecdotal evidence, expert opinions, drug company promotions, and their clinical experience rather than on developments in clinical research and scientific evaluations of new methods of diagnostic, treatment, management or service delivery.

Perhaps because evidence-based practice at McMaster University was integrated into medical education at pre and post-qualification, impressive advances were made in developing the dissemination and understanding of research into clinical practice. Amongst these advances were randomised trials of teaching methods for research-appraisal skills to undergraduates, the use of information technology to access research information to inform clinical decision-making, the development of abstracting, appraising and disseminating clinical research to clinicians, and the adaptation of statistical methods to relate more directly to clinical significance.

Recent health care policy shows clearly how evidence-based practice has been supported in the UK National Health Service. Clinical audit was introduced to the NHS by the 1989 White Paper, *Working for patients*. In 1991 the NHS appointed a director of research and development, and published a research and development strategy which included support for the UK Cochrane Centre, the NHS Centre for Reviews and Dissemination, the Health Technology Assessment Programme and programmes of research in specific clinical areas. The 1992 White Paper, *Health of the Nation*, set national targets for improvements in key health areas and required the health service to increase the knowledge base of clinical practice and cost-effectiveness; and the 1993 White Paper, *Realising our Potential*, again emphasised the importance of linking research to practical issues and the dissemination of research findings. More recently, the 1997 White Paper, *The new NHS: modern, dependable*, refers to the establishment of a National Institute for Clinical Effectiveness (NICE).

The process of evidence-based practice

The development of evidence-based medicine was thus based on three principles:

(1) Doctors must be taught how to interpret and use research findings.
(2) Doctors must be helped to use research to inform practice throughout their careers.
(3) Research findings must be disseminated to doctors in more efficient ways.

Within the context of evidence-based medicine the roles of researchers and clinicians are changed. Thus, clinicians are defined as consumers of research, a subtle restatement of the role of research in practice. In this formulation, there are clear, mutual responsibilities of clinicians and researchers; clinicians need to develop skills to evaluate research (critical appraisal skills) and keep up to date with research findings, and researchers need to develop methods of disseminating research effectively to clinicians.

Evidence-based practice is seen as consisting of five explicit steps:

(1) First, the clinician, faced with a patient or group of patients, constructs a specific question concerning their care. This could relate to the

diagnosis of the problem, the prognosis or likely outcome of the problem, the most effective treatments and their possible side-effects, or the best method of delivering services to meet patients' needs.

(2) The second stage consists of finding, as efficiently as possible, the best evidence to answer the clinical question.

(3) Third, the clinician evaluates the evidence for its validity and usefulness.

(4) Fourth, the results are applied to the specific patient or group of patients.

(5) Finally, the outcome of the intervention is evaluated.

Clinical questions

Although evidence-based medicine is frequently associated with the evaluation of treatment methods, clinical questions within the context of evidence-based medicine may involve any aspect of the clinical encounter. Thus clinical questions may concern the etiology or cause of a problem, diagnosis (or assessment), prognosis, economics and costs, treatment methods, preventative interventions or methods of service delivery and organisation. The identification of clinical questions is seen as a core requirement of evidence-based practice. Sackett *et al.* (1996) describe the development of clinical questions which emerge in the light of clinical findings from the interview and any physical examinations.

Clinical questions have four components. The first of these is the patient or problem. The patient is described in relation to the medical problem for which they seek help along with any relevant demographic features. It may, for example, be important to clarify that a patient is a child, or is elderly, or in the case of some medical conditions, that they are male or female. The second component is the clinical action to be taken. In a question relating to treatment this would be the identified treatment which is being considered; in a question relating to diagnosis this would be a specific test or procedure. The third component is the contrast or comparison action, the alternative treatment or intervention, or the standard diagnostic test. Finally, the clinical question should identify a clear outcome or set of outcomes against which the action can be evaluated. This might include mortality or morbidity in treatment questions, and accuracy in a diagnostic question. Examples of complete clinical questions are shown in Box 2.2.

Finding the evidence

Having identified a specific clinical question the next step within evidence-based practice is to find relevant evidence relating to the question. A core problem related to the identification of evidence is that for most clinicians

> **Box 2.2: Examples of clinical questions**
>
> **Treatment**
>
> Patient: In **children with depression**
>
> Clinical action: does **cognitive therapy,**
>
> Comparison: when compared **with tricyclic antidepressants** alone,
>
> Outcomes: lead to **fewer symptoms** of depression?
>
> **Diagnosis**
>
> Patient: In **non-symptomatic adults**
>
> Clinical action: does **routine screening** for colorectal cancer
>
> Comparison: compared **with no routine screening**
>
> Outcomes: **increase diagnosis** and lead to **reduced mortality?**

the sheer weight of evidence reported in research journals is overwhelming. Because of this huge amount of information, doctors have traditionally relied upon a limited range of sources to update their knowledge. These include promotional materials distributed by pharmaceutical companies, training events, attendance at conferences, discussions with colleagues, professional (i.e. non-academic journals), and textbooks. Evidence-based medicine practitioners argue that each of these sources is likely to be seriously biased and they have therefore developed a range of methods which take advantage of the increasing accessibility of information technologies.

There are now numerous sources of medical information. These include unselected databases of relevant academic journals (e.g. MEDLINE, PsychLit, BIDS). In addition there are an ever increasing number of evidence-based resources, including websites (e.g. OXAMWEB); CD-ROMS which highlight high-quality clinical studies (e.g. *Best Evidence, Cochrane Library*); evidence-based guidelines developed by professional bodies; as well as a new range of journals which provide up-to-date summaries of high-quality research (e.g. *Evidence-Based Medicine, Evidence-Based Mental Health*). For further details of all these resources see Box 2.1.

Traditional literature reviews using unselected databases (e.g. MEDLINE) frequently result in the identification of many possible references of interest (Greenhalgh 1997). Thus, for example, a search on MEDLINE using the terms 'depression' and 'children' results in a list of 718 articles. Similarly a MEDLINE search from 1996, using the terms 'screening' and 'colorectal cancer' results in a list of 507 references. Such abundance of information may be required in some circumstances, but in clinical settings is likely to be unhelpful and overwhelming.

Evidence-based medicine provides two solutions to this practical problem. The first solution is more demanding of the clinician's skills and time. The clinician must learn how to be selective in searching the literature, and having been selective must apply the principles of critical appraisal (see following section) to decide if the results of the study are relevant to his or her clinical question. The second solution is more simple. Using evidence-based resources, the clinician can search within a more limited database in which research is included only if it is of high quality *and* clinically relevant. Using the same clinical questions again with evidence-based resources provides a much more limited but potentially clinically useful list of relevant research.

Critical appraisal

This range of evidence-based resources provides specific information about clinical research to doctors and other health professionals. Whilst they aim to remove most of the work involved in identifying clinically relevant research they are, however, only a partial solution. An integral part of evidence-based medicine, therefore, consists of evaluating the evidence that is found. The core skill of critical appraisal forms the third part of the evidence-based process. Critical appraisal, in the context of evidence-based medicine, consists of two stages in which the research is appraised for validity and clinical importance.

The first stage in the process is to establish if the research is valid. In this context, validity refers to the extent to which the results of the research are likely to be free from bias. Thus specific methodological criteria are used to evaluate research studies. In the context of EBM, clinically relevant research is classified into the following types of research:

- etiology
- therapuetics
- diagnosis
- prognosis
- quality improvement
- economic evaluation.

Specific methodological criteria have been identified for the evaluation of each of these different categories of research. Thus for example, studies of prevention or treatment are considered valid if they have the following characteristics: random allocation of participants to comparison groups; follow-up of at least 80% of those entering the study; outcome measures of known or probable clinical importance; and analysis of data which is consistent with the design. Studies of prognosis are considered valid if they have an inception cohort (i.e. individuals in the study enter the study either at the onset of the disorder or at a uniform point in the development of the disorder), if at least 80% of patients in the study are followed-up, and if the data analysis is consistent with the study design.

Although evidence-based medicine is concerned with a wide range of clinical questions and study designs, much attention has been drawn to questions and study designs concerned with the evaluation of treatment methods. Within this category of research the best known methodology promoted by evidence-based medicine is the randomised controlled trial (RCT). The RCT is frequently cited as the 'gold standard' method of assessing the efficacy of treatment methods. The core feature of an RCT is the random allocation of all potential participants to the control or to the experimental treatment. Random allocation to conditions, regardless of the personal preference of the patients, the expectations of their doctors, and of any other personal characteristics and qualities, ensures that all sources of bias are distributed at random between the control and experimental groups.

The RCT is generally accepted to be the best, though not the only, method of evaluating treatment efficacy. Quantitative reviews of more than one RCT study by meta-analysis are deemed to provide the optimal summary of current knowledge regarding treatment methods. Guyatt *et al.* (1995) outlined a hierarchy of methods for evaluating treatment effects:

(1)   Systematic reviews and meta-analyses.
(2)   Randomised controlled trials with definitive results.
(3)   Randomised controlled trials with non-definitive results.
(4)   Cohort studies.
(5)   Case-control studies.
(6)   Cross-sectional studies.
(7)   Case reports.

Additional methodological features are also desirable in evaluations of therapy or prevention and are generally required to minimise bias. Thus, for example RCTs are ideally double blind, in that patient and doctor are both unaware to which of the two conditions (control or experimental) the patient has been allocated. Similarly, the assessor of clinical outcome (if not the patient or doctor) should also be blind to treatment allocation. RCT studies must follow up their patients in order to assess the relative effects of the experimental and control conditions. In order to ensure that this follow-up is relatively unbiased a threshold of 80% follow-up is frequently set.

Randomisation of patients to treatments is sometimes not possible for ethical or practical reasons. This might occur in the treatment of a rare condition where insufficient numbers of patients are available for a trial. In such circumstances alternative methods of evaluation may be necessary and in some areas of clinical practice, well-controlled experimental case studies are the preferred method of assessing the efficacy of a new treatment.

Thus, in the case of a therapy study, criteria relating to validity include the random assignment of patients to treatment conditions, high rates of follow-up of patients and blind assessment of outcomes. If studies are valid, the second stage of critical appraisal is to establish if the results of the study are clinically important.

The concept of clinical importance is used to replace the more traditional concept of statistical significance. In medical research it is common to use dichotomous categories to assess the outcome of an intervention. Examples of such dichotomous categories include the presence or absence of a specific diagnostic category, harmful events like side-effects or re-admission to hospital, or more simply whether the patient is alive or dead. Statistical tests are used to evaluate the likelihood that an observed difference in outcomes between treatment groups is due to the play of chance. Thus, arbitrary levels of significance are used which indicate that the differences between treatments are likely to occur by chance less than 5% of the time, or less than 1% of the time. Statistical tests, however, do not help interpret the clinical importance of the difference in outcome. In evidence-based practice different methods of estimating clinical importance of research results are used. These include the number needed to treat (NNT) and the number needed to harm (NNH). NNT and NNH translate the results of an intervention into figures which indicate how many patients would have to be treated with the treatment method in order to bring about one good outcome or one harmful outcome. A worked example of an NNT calculation is shown in Box 2.3. Further detailed information on the use of NNT and NNH can be found in Sackett *et al* (1997).

Application to individual patients

The aim of evidence-based medicine is to bring research into clinical practice and the fourth stage of the process involves applying the research findings to the care and management of individual patients. Patients who have participated in clinical trials frequently differ from those seen in routine practice and the clinician must make a judgement about how well the results of a trial will generalise beyond the trial itself. In addition to considering how applicable trial results are likely to be to individual patients, the clinician is also required to consider if the treatment is consistent with the patient's values and expectations. If a depressed patient is reluctant to take a course of antidepressant medication then even the most efficacious drug regime will not be suitable for them.

The application of clinical research to the care of individual patients presents a core challenge for evidence-based practice. This is because well-designed experimental studies are constructed so as to exclude as many

---

Box 2.3: Worked example of numbers needed to treat (NNT)

The following example illustrates the method of calculating the NNT.

In a study by Kendall *et al.* (1997) 94 children aged 9–13 years with a primary anxiety disorder were allocated either to cognitive–behaviour therapy (CBT) or to a waiting list control group. At the end of treatment 53% of the children who had received therapy no longer met diagnostic criteria for anxiety. Only 6% of children in the waiting list control group no longer met diagnostic criteria for anxiety.

These figures give us the data necessary to calculate the NNT:
First it is necessary to calculate the ABI (absolute benefits increase). This is the absolute arithmetic difference in event rates of a positive outcome. The ABI is calculated by subtracting the event rate in the control group (CER) from the event rate in the experimental group (EER).

$$ABI = (EER - CER) = (53\% - 6\%) = 47\%$$

The NNT is calculated as $\frac{1}{ABI}$ and denotes the number of patients who must receive the experimental treatment to create on additional improved outcome in comparison with the control treatment. Thus the NNT in the Kendall *et al.* study is $\frac{1}{0.47}$ = 2.13. This is conventionally rounded up to the next highest integer, in this case 3. Thus an NNT of 3 indicates that 3 children with anxiety disorder need to be treated with CBT in order to achieve one more child free of the anxiety disorder compared with the control group.

---

possible sources of bias and of confounding as is practical. This process serves to increase the internal validity of the study, that is, the extent to which the results of an experiment can be attributed to the specific intervention that is to be tested. In all experiments there is a trade-off between internal and external validity. External validity refers to the extent to which the results of a study can be generalised to other settings. Unfortunately, the characteristics of research design that strengthen internal validity almost always weaken the study's external validity. Thus, for example, research designs will often call for the careful recruitment of patients to studies. During assessment for the trial various exclusion criteria may apply. These criteria vary across studies but common exclusion criteria include co-morbid disorders, inability to speak or write English fluently, chronicity of the disorder, unclear diagnostic status, or receipt of other forms of treatment. Other features of a study which may reduce external validity include the setting (teaching versus non-teaching hospital), the clinicians (research aware versus research unaware), and the inclusion of additional follow-up assessments (Shadish *et al.* 1997).

In addition to these methodological issues, the results of experimental clinical trials almost always report the overall effects of the intervention. Within this overall result there may be considerable variation in the responses of individual patients to treatment. Thus, whilst some improve, others may stay the same, and others may deteriorate. The majority of clinical trials do not attempt to identify sub-groups of patients for whom the treatment may be effective, ineffective or harmful.

The application of research findings to individual patients inevitably relies on clinical judgement. Within evidence-based medicine two questions can be formulated to help clinicians make this judgement. First, the clinician must judge if their patient is broadly similar to those patients included in the trial, and what the probable benefit to the patient may be. Sackett *et al.* (1997) suggest that the emphasis of the clinician should not be on considering whether each individual patient would meet the inclusion criteria for the trial, but rather on whether the individual patient is so different from those in the trial that the results could not possibly apply. The probable benefits to the patient can be estimated by reference to the NNT. Small NNTs indicate that benefit is likely, large NNTs indicate that benefit is less likely. Second, the clinician is expected to consider the treatment option in relation to the patient's own values and preferences. If these are not consistent with those necessary for compliance with the treatment then however large the potential benefits may be, the treatment is unlikely to be helpful.

Evaluating the impact of care

The process of evaluation is central to evidence-based medicine. Clinicians using evidence-based medicine are encouraged to evaluate continually their own performance in relation to their use of evidence-based medicine and are encouraged to evaluate the validity and importance of clinically relevant research (Sackett *et al.* 1997). Less often discussed is the extent to which evidence-based medicine clinicians are encouraged to ask the question 'Is this treatment working for this patient?' Because most methods of treatment may have no effects, or negative effects for some patients, it is important that outcomes for individual patients are monitored, and that treatment is adjusted accordingly. Moreover, in clinical practice, it is this question concerning the responsiveness of an individual patient that is likely to confront the clinician on a daily basis.

Clinicians may monitor patients' outcomes on an individual basis or as part of a service-wide audit process. This aspect of evidence-based medicine has the potential to overcome some of the problems of making clinical decisions on the basis of RCT evidence alone. As described above, there are a number of methodological characteristics of RCT which make the translation of RCT results to clinical practice difficult. A distinction can be drawn between *efficacy* studies (usually RCTs) which can demonstrate the potential benefits of a treatment method under experimental conditions; and *effectiveness* studies which can demonstrate the benefits of a treatment method in normal 'real-world settings' (Hoagwood *et al.* 1995).

Wade *et al.* (1998) reported an effectiveness study of a psychological treatment for panic disorder. RCT evidence suggested that cognitive–behaviour therapy was beneficial (e.g. Barlow *et al.* 1989; Margraf *et al.* 1993) and Wade *et al.* (1998) examined the outcomes of CBT for panic disorder in a US community mental health centre. Compared with patients who participated in previous RCTs, patients in the Wade *et al.* study tended to be younger, had fewer years of education, were more likely to be taking medication for their psychological problems, reported more severe distress, and had more co-morbid disorders. Despite these differences between the samples the results of the Wade *et al.* study were similar to those reported in the RCT studies; 87% of treatment completers were panic-free at the end of treatment.

The results of the Wade *et al.* study indicate that psychological treatment may be beneficial to anxious clients in a community setting. However, efficacy studies are rarely conducted and rarely reported in the research literature and other efficacy studies within mental health have been less encouraging. Thus for example, Weisz *et al.* (1995) contrasted the results of four meta-analyses (comprising over 200 individual controlled studies) of psychotherapy for children with a smaller number of 'clinically representative studies'. They observed that the clinically representative studies showed more modest effects of psychotherapy than had the meta-analyses and suggested that the characteristics of controlled research in psychotherapy resulted in misleading and overly positive outcomes.

Clearly the clinical utility of RCT evidence cannot be assessed on the basis of these few studies in the specific context of psychological therapies. However, the results of these studies do illustrate that the results of RCTs may not always transfer easily to uncontrolled clinical settings. Thus if clinicians are to make confident estimates of the benefits of treatments for their individual patients there is a need for effectiveness as well as efficacy research within EBM.

Problems of evidence-based medicine

Evidence-based medicine has been described as revolutionary and as challenging traditional expert-based authoritarian management in medicine (Grayson 1997). Inevitably, perhaps, evidence-based medicine has met with a degree of hostility, scepticism, and from some, outright rejection (e.g. Polychronis *et al.* 1996a, 1996b). Concerns about evidence-based medicine appear to fall into three main categories. First is the concern that evidence-based medicine provides a structure within which to ration health care. Second is the fear that evidence-based medicine threatens the professional autonomy of individual doctors. Third is the objection that evidence-based medicine presents a distorted and partial view of science and rejects much that is central to the scientific method.

Rationing of health care

Of particular concern, is the link that has been made between evidence-based medicine and the rationing of health care. The link between evidence-based medicine and the efficient use of resources in health care dates back to the early writings of Archie Cochrane. Evidence-based medicine aims to promote the most effective care of patients. The effects of evidence-based medicine can therefore, and sometime do, highlight common methods of treatment which appear to be ineffective or harmful. Few clinicians or patients would probably argue that ineffective or harmful treatment should be provided by health services. However, it is also clear that many, if not most medical (and surgical) interventions, have never been formally evaluated, and certainly not in a way that would meet the stringent requirements of randomised controlled trials as established by Cochrane. What does this mean for the practice of medicine: could evidence-based medicine be used as a way of prohibiting expensive treatments which have not been formally evaluated? More importantly, could treatments be prohibited for all patients, if they are effective for only a minority of patients?

The development of evidence-based practice in the UK has been directly supported by government policy. Grayson suggests that:

> 'evidence-based medicine with its emphasis on eradicating useless or wasteful practices and concentrating on those which deliver the best outcome has enormous attractions as a tool for targeting scarce resources, and is fully in line with the commitment of both major political parties to the promotion of efficiency and monitoring of performance'.
>
> (Grayson 1997: 19)

Sackett *et al.* (1997) have strenuously refuted the idea that evidence-based medicine should be used to reduce costs or to ration expensive treatments. Clinicians using evidence-based medicine should use their clinical experience and judgement combined with their knowledge of research to decide the best treatment of individual patients. At this level, considerations of cost do not apply and the focus of concern is the well-being of the individual patient. More problematic, however, is that specific clinical services may be purchased or decommissioned by purchasers on the basis of effectiveness and/or cost (Gray 1997).

Limits to professional autonomy

Linked with concerns that evidence-based medicine may be used to inform decisions about rationing health care services, some clinicians have raised objections to the constraints that evidence-based medicine may place on the autonomy of professionals in clinical decision-making (e.g. Hampton 1997). In part, resistance to evidence-based medicine may be based on a reluctance to devalue traditional authority structures within medicine and health care more generally. Grayson (1997) suggests that some doctors argue that evidence-based medicine fails to acknowledge that medical care and medical decision-making often take place in conditions of considerable uncertainty and that in such conditions, the art of medicine and of health care is as important as the science.

An additional concern for some clinicians is that evidence-based medicine can only be effective in clinical settings where good quality evidence is available; thus in areas of health care which are not well researched evidence-based medicine has little to offer and may stifle innovative new treatments and other developments. For example, some areas of medicine (e.g. hematology, neurology, general practice) and other areas of health care (e.g. nursing, occupational therapy and physiotherapy) have been poorly served by the research community and thus have little research on which to base their practice. Thus the stringent implementation of evidence-based practice in these areas of health care may threaten core services to vulnerable populations.

A *distorted version of science*

Evidence-based medicine developed from a particular view of the use of science in medicine. Some commentators suggest that the development of evidence-based medicine threatens to constrain other, equally valid, scientifically based research and promotes an overly narrow range of research methodologies. For example, within evidence-based medicine the role of the experimental single case study is demoted to a fall-back strategy for use only when superior forms of evidence are unavailable (Sackett *et al.* 1997). Within this world-view the experimental case study is very much a poor relation to the RCT. However, this view of the single case experiment fails to acknowledge that such a research strategy may be the most appropriate in developing new methods of treatment, or where other service or clinical constraints make the use of RCT impractical or unethical.

Other concerns about the application of evidence-based medicine, particularly beyond areas of clinical medicine, relate to questions about the validity of categorical diagnostic systems, the use of dichotomous outcome measures which provide only a partial reflection of clinical outcomes, and the limited range of outcome measures that are selected for use in RCTs. Within mental health, for example, there are well-rehearsed arguments concerning the validity of diagnostic classification and the reification of such diagnostic categories. Similarly, outcomes typically used in RCTs of obstetric procedures rarely incorporate psychological or quality-of-life variables for the patient, and focus on a relatively restricted range of physiological variables.

Another area of concern in relation to evidence-based medicine is the overwhelming focus on *quantitative* research methods and their related questions, a concern raised by a number of authors in this book. Thus, although at the heart of evidence-based medicine is the care of individual patients, and the integration of research evidence with patient preferences and values, *qualitative* research – which may have much to say about the values, preferences and experiences of patients (and of their doctors) – has been largely ignored. There are clear signs that the status of qualitative research within evidence-based medicine is changing. Criteria for the appraisal of qualitative research have been developed, and continue to be developed (e.g. Greenhalgh 1997). Some of the evidence-based journals include or plan to include qualitative research, and there appears to be an increasing acknowledgement within evidence-based medicine that the principle which determines what kind of research is of value is dictated by the specific clinical question. The introduction of qualitative research methods within evidence-based medicine marks a significant shift in its development. The extent to which this shift will influence the core values of evidence-based medicine is so far unclear.

Conclusion

Although evidence-based medicine has had a remarkable impact on health policy in the UK its introduction has not been universally welcomed and the integration of evidence-based medicine principles within medicine and within the wider spheres of professional practice has been patchy. As is implied by the title of this book the impact of evidence-based medicine has been felt far beyond the discipline of medicine and many of the principles and methods of evidence-based medicine have been transferred to other areas of professional practice. Inevitably this transfer is not always straightforward, particularly where the underlying principles of the profession differ from the underlying principles of evidence-based medicine.

References

Antman E., Lau J., Kupeltruck B., Mosteller F. & Chalmers I. (1992) A comparison of the results of meta-analyses of randomised controlled trials and recommendations of clinical experts. *Journal of the American Medical Association*, **268**, 240–48.

Barlow D., Craske M., Cerny J. & Klosko J. (1989) Behavioral treatment of panic disorder. *Behavior Therapy*, **20**, 261–82.

Cochrane A. (1972) *Effectiveness and Efficiency: Random Reflection on Health Services.* Nuffield Provincial Hospitals Trust, London.

Grayson L. (1997) *Evidence-Based Medicine*. British Library, London.

Gray J.A.M. (1997) *Evidence-Based Healthcare: How to Make Health Policy and Management Decisions*. Churchill Livingstone, London.

Greenhalgh T. (1997) *How to Read a Paper: The Basics of Evidence-Based Medicine*. BMJ Publishing Group, London.

Guyatt G., Sackett D., Sinclair J., Hayward R., Cook D. & Cook R. (1995) Users' Guides to the Medical Literature 9. A method for grading health-care recommendations. *Journal of the American Medical Association*, **274**, 1800–804.

Hampton J.R. (1997) Evidence-based medicine, practice variations and clinical freedom. *Journal of Evaluation in Clinical Practice*, **3**, 123–31.

Hoagwood K., Hibbs E., Brent D. & Jensen P. (1995) Introduction to the Special Section – Efficacy and effectiveness in studies of child and adolescent psychotherapy. *Journal of Consulting and Clinical Psychology*, **63**, 683–7.

Kendall P., Flannery-Schroeder E. & Panichelli-Mindel S. (1997) Therapy for youths with anxiety disorders: a second randomized clinical trial. *Journal of Consulting and Clinical Psychology*, **65**, 366–80.

Margraf J., Barlow D., Clark D. & Telch M. (1993) Psychological treatment of panic – work in progress on outcome, active ingredients, and follow-up. *Behaviour Research and Therapy*, **31**, 1–8.

Polychronis A., Miles A. & Bentley D.P. (1996a) Evidence-based medicine: Reference? Dogma? Neologism? New orthodoxy? *Journal of Evaluation in Clinical Practice*, **2**, 1–3.

Polychronis A., Miles A. & Bentley D.P. (1996b) The protagonists of EBM: arrogant, seductive and controversial. *Journal of Evaluation in Clinical Practice*, **2**, 9–12.

Ramsey P.G., Garline J.D., Inue T.S., Larsen E., Logerfo J., Norun J. & Wenrich M. (1991) Changes over time in the knowledge base of practising internists. *Journal of the American Medical Association*, **266**, 1103–7.

Sackett D.L., Richardson W.S., Rosenberg W. & Haynes R.B. (1997) *Evidence-Based Medicine: How to Practice and Teach EBM*. Churchill Livingstone, New York.

Sackett D.L., Haynes R.B., Guyatt G.H. & Tugwell P. (1991) *Clinical Epidemiology: A Basic Science for Clinical Medicine* (2nd edition). Little Brown, Boston.

Shadish W.R., Matt G.E., Navarro A.M., Siegle G., Crits-Cristoph P., *et al.* (1997) Evidence that therapy works in clinically representative conditions. *Journal of Consulting and Clinical Psychology*, **65**, 355–65.

Wade W.A., Treat T.A. & Stuart G.L. (1998) Transporting an empirically supported treatment for panic disorder to a service clinic setting: a benchmarking strategy. *Journal of Consulting and Clinical Psychology*, **66**, 231–9.

Weisz J.R., Donenberg G.R., Han S.S. & Weiss B. (1995) Bridging the gap between laboratory and clinic in child and adolescent psychotherapy. *Journal of Consulting and Clinical Psychology*, **63**, 688–701.

Chapter 3

Evidence-Based Practice in General Practice and Primary Care

Toby Lipman

Introduction

The majority of health interventions in the UK are delivered by primary care. It is the first port of call for most individuals when they perceive themselves to be ill, or require services such as contraception, health screening or immunisation. In the classic job definition of general practice the general practitioner '... accepts the responsibility for making an initial decision on every problem his patient may present to him, consulting with specialists when he thinks it appropriate to do so' (Royal College of General Practitioners 1969). Although primary care is often thought of as general practice, general practitioners (GPs) are also members of primary health care teams (Mackichan 1976). These consist of practice nurses, district nurses and health visitors and may include dieticians, physiotherapists, counsellors, pharmacists and psychiatric nurses, as well as essential non-clinical staff such as managers, secretaries and receptionists. They are state-funded, and the cost of funding large primary health care teams may exceed £1,000,000 per annum.

Some primary care is delivered outside the primary health care team – by school nurses, optometrists, dentists, community pediatricians and others (including hospital casualty departments) – but it would require an entire book rather than one chapter to describe the potential of evidence-based practice for all of these. I will therefore discuss them within the context of the primary health care team, focusing on primary health care in the UK. It should, however, also be recognised that an international community of primary care clinicians and researchers has developed over the years, and that there have been important developments in primary care in many countries in Europe (particularly Holland), in North America, Australia and New Zealand, and many other countries.

Although most health care contacts take place in primary care, three times as much money is spent on secondary (hospital/specialist) and tertiary (super-specialist) care compared to primary care (NHS Executive

1996) (see Box 3.1). One of primary care's most important roles is therefore as gatekeeper to the secondary and tertiary sectors. This is made possible by the referral system and the system of patient registration (Coulter 1992; Oswald 1992). The overall referral rate has been reported as 47 per 1000 consultations although it varies widely between different GPs (Royal College of General Practitioners 1992; Fertig *et al.* 1993). Almost all individuals in the UK are registered with a local practice. Their medical records are kept at the practice and referral to a specialist is possible only through the general practitioner. Patients are entitled to change to a different practice if they wish (and must do so if they move outside the practice area) but they may not be registered with more than one practice at a time. If they change practice, their medical record follows them (and is perhaps the only aspect of the Welfare State envisaged by the 1945 Labour government which can truly be said to stay with individuals 'from cradle to grave').

Box 3.1: NHS gross expenditure 1995–96 (estimate) – England

	£
• Hospital and community health services capital	1.9bn
• Hospital and community health services current	23.6bn
• Family health services current non-cash limited	8.2bn
• Central health and miscellaneous services	0.6bn
• Department administration	0.3bn
Total	34.7bn

Source: Department of Health

From the 1960s, general practice evolved into primary care, with expansion of the range of services provided to patients and the development of the primary health care team. Practice nurses were employed by GPs to fulfil roles covering, amongst others, cervical cytology, chronic care, well-patient screening. District nurses, health visitors, secretaries, practice managers, social workers, physiotherapists, counsellors and others joined the team; practices became larger; GPs such as Geoffrey Marsh advocated the idea of efficient practice, in which the GP was seen as the leader of a large and diverse multidisciplinary team (Marsh 1991). The position and status of other professions within primary care remains sharply differentiated from and subservient to that of GPs, and this is still an unresolved dilemma. Although we talk and write of primary care and primary health care teams, most change has been initiated by and owned by GPs or the government. The other professions within the team have less power and are often directly employed by GPs.

At the same time, criticism of GPs with poor standards mounted. Donald Irvine (1985) wrote 'let there be no mistake, Government and society mean what they say – they intend to sort out our standards of care in their own way unless we show more inclination and more energy to do so ourselves'. (Sir Donald Irvine was Chairman of Council of the Royal College of General Practitioners from 1982 to 1985 and is currently President of the General Medical Council.) This message was unpalatable to and resented by much of the profession. Many GPs were also aggrieved that, when the NHS reforms were implemented in 1990, they appeared to reflect much of the RCGPs agenda from the preceding decade. The college hierarchy was accused of secretly conniving with the government and some GPs were vitriolic in their criticism. Some resigned from the college, and it has taken the college several years since then to re-establish credibility with much of the profession.

The reforms themselves were based on the idea of an internal market in the NHS, on the assumption that GPs would become purchasers and managers of care, that performance could be improved by setting targets, and that business methods would inevitably raise standards. The idea that GPs should be entrepreneurs was not universally supported. There was 'a feeling that politicians and health service planners are seeking to place general practice at the centre of the NHS without properly understanding the essential transactions of its discipline' (Heath 1995).

Free market economics also led to an increasing disparity between rich and poor, and widespread disruption of patterns of life established over generations (Hutton 1995). Throughout the 1980s and 1990s, primary care, particularly in inner city areas, witnessed and tried to cope with the health consequences of free market economics (Widgery 1991).

Another consequence of free market philosophy was consumerism, the idea that patients have become consumers of the health care services of which the NHS is a provider. It is hard to think of patients with terminal cancer, heart failure or dementia as 'consumers', or equate what primary health care teams do with what supermarkets or travel agents do. Moreover, whereas in the commercial world every extra customer is a source of income, in primary health care the resources for providing care to a defined population are fixed, and every extra consultation is equivalent to a cost. It has been suggested that 'while the thrust towards empowering the patient is a welcome redress for past paternalism, it has had the unintended consequence of marginalising the doctor's view' (Fairhurst & May 1995).

These changes have made primary care a troubled arena. Morale among many GPs is low and recruitment of GP registrars (formerly called trainees) is falling (Rowsell *et al.* 1995). Perhaps the overriding feeling is that the changes have been driven by political ideology and economic theories, rather than by evidence or pragmatic considerations, and that the views of professionals within primary care have been ignored (unless they happened to coincide with the government's ideological position).

The new Labour government has lost no time in making further changes to primary care. Fundholding, in which GP 'fundholders' received a budget with which to purchase secondary care services, community care (district nurses and health visitors) and drugs, and in which planned savings could be re-invested in further services to patients (such as physiotherapy, consultant clinics in the surgery, and so on) was abolished from 1 April 1999. Instead all the practices in a locality (typically 70 000 to 120 000 patients) will join a 'primary care group' (PCG) to commission secondary care and community services. This is supposed to be more equitable, to reduce the administrative burdens associated with fundholding, and to form the basis of a 'primary care-led' NHS. However, many GPs are wary, and feel that PCGs may prove as bureaucratic as fundholding, while reducing their cherished professional independence. In their most developed form ('Stage 4'), PCGs will be accountable to health authorities for commissioning secondary care services, and providing community services (Secretary of State for Health 1997). It is hard to see how this organisational structure can be compatible with GPs' status as independent contractors. The success or otherwise of PCGs may depend on how well the transition of GPs from self-employed partners in small businesses to salaried employees of primary care groups is managed. Logical (and even desirable) though this may be in terms of the overall effectiveness of primary care, it is likely to meet fierce resistance in some quarters.

In addition to organisational change, the government has, for the first time, put in place measures to ensure clinical effectiveness and quality assurance. The National Institute of Clinical Evidence (NICE) will 'give new coherence and prominence to information about clinical and cost-effectiveness'; at local level, NHS Trusts and PCGs are required to embrace 'clinical governance' to ensure that services provided to patients are of the highest possible quality (Secretary of State for Health 1997). The concept of clinical governance explicitly requires that 'evidence-based practice is in day-to-day use with the infrastructure to support it' (along with other quality assurance measures such as clinical audit). However, as a detailed discussion document on clinical governance observes, 'the professional skills required to practice evidence-based health care are thought to be not widely available' (NHSE North Thames Region 1998). At present it appears that clinical governance is likely to follow a quality assurance model, based on standard-setting, clinical audit, risk management and organisational development, with an assumption that evidence-based practice by individual clinicians will play only a minor role.

The research and practice background

The Royal College of Physicians was founded in 1518, the United Company of Barber Surgeons in 1540 (becoming the Royal College of Surgeons in

1800) and the Society of Apothecaries in 1617. The College of General Practitioners (later the Royal College of General Practitioners) was not founded until November 1952, 434 years after the Royal College of Physicians. During the late nineteenth to early twentieth centuries, general practice had gradually evolved into a form which we would recognise today, although the distinction between general practitioners and specialists was not formalised until the formation of the NHS in 1948. Before this, general practitioners often also held hospital posts and consultants often dabbled in general practice.

The founders of the College aimed to improve standards in general practice and to raise its status. This was an uphill task, as medical schools were (and largely remain) attached to teaching hospitals, whose consultants dominated the medical curriculum, often speaking in disparaging terms of general practice and general practitioners. It was assumed that the brightest students would enter a career in hospital medicine, and those who 'fell off the ladder', in Lord Moran's phrase, would fall into general practice. These attitudes are far from extinct even today (Petchey *et al.* 1997).

Traditionally, general practitioners learned medicine from and deferred to consultants, whose expertise and knowledge was regarded as authoritative. A good general practitioner was one who most thoroughly attended to the advice and superior knowledge of hospital specialists. Sackett and his colleagues describe this attitude as an 'abdication to authority' and observe that 'to base your treatment of commonly encountered problems on the advice of some "expert" who publishes treatment recommendations but no supporting evidence puts you on a par with the barefoot doctor. After all, it was these same experts who advocated turpentine stopes and leeches' (Sackett *et al.* 1991). This argument for evidence-based practice might also apply to the condition of general practice before the foundation of its college.

The College set out to encourage original research in general practice by general practitioners, to establish vocational training for general practitioners, and to establish an academic base for general practice. That meaningful research could be done in general practice had been established before the Second World War by outstanding individuals such as William Pickles, who carried out epidemiological research in his practice in Wensleydale (Pickles 1939). Julian Tudor Hart, who qualified in 1952, set out to undertake a lifetime's research in a single-handed practice in Wales, convinced that medical research ought to be carried out in the settings in which patients lived and worked (Hart 1974). However, in 1952 there was not one university department of general practice, so doing research and developing vocational training was an act of faith driven by 'a passionate belief in the future of general practice' (Swift 1982).

One of the most influential early strands in general practice research was initiated not by a GP, but by a psychoanalyst, Michael Balint (Balint 1964). His work gave general practice its own specialty – the consultation. Much research on doctor–patient interactions followed, and both the understanding of the consultation and Balint's non-directive teaching methods found their way into the curriculum of vocational training for general practice and the wider culture of general practice (Byrne & Long 1976; Pendleton *et al.* 1984; Royal College of General Practitioners 1972). Throughout the 1960s and 1970s, vocational training schemes expanded and in 1981 it became a legal requirement for general practitioners to have undergone an approved three-year course of vocational training before being allowed to practice as an unrestricted principal. The consultation remains central to vocational training, and the educational process by which the findings of this body of research are translated into clinical practice has become increasingly sophisticated (Neighbour 1987). Although general practice vocational training schemes have also tried to encourage registrars to develop an interest in research, trainers often do not have the expertise to support this, and the demands of learning how to be a competent general practitioner leave little time for the extra work that research entails (Buckley 1995).

Balint's work was qualitative, conducted and put into practice at a time when quantitative research was the dominant paradigm in medicine. General practice and primary care deal with patients who may or may not have diseases, rather than with diseases which have patients attached to them. Research in primary care is therefore concerned with a multiplicity of questions, which include practice organisation, the primary–secondary interface, diagnosis and treatment of disease, epidemiology, prescribing, patient satisfaction, approaches to consulting and many others. Qualitative methods were always appropriate to the primary care setting, although methodology has matured and become more sophisticated in recent years (Britten *et al.* 1995). However, researchers are ready to use whatever research methodology is appropriate to the research question and both quantitative and qualitative methods are used (Box 3.2).

Different methods may be used to investigate aspects of the same topic. For example, John Fry recorded his own referral patterns, then set out a research agenda up to the present day by asking 'what are the habits of family doctors in referring patients to hospital and why do these habits vary so much?' (Fry 1959). Other studies might be very elaborate, involving complex statistical analysis to correct for confounding factors, in order to demonstrate that variation in referral rates is a genuine phenomenon (Cummins *et al.* 1981), or use expert panels to assess the quality of referrals (Knottnerus *et al.* 1990). In one study, rate of elective admission to hospitals was used as a proxy measure of appropriateness of referral – practices with higher referral rates also had higher admission rates (Coulter *et al.* 1990). A qualitative study using semi-structured interviews found that high referrers

Box 3.2: Qualitative and quantitative research questions

	Qualitative	*Quantitative*
Descriptive		
Typical questions	What is going on here?	How many?
	What is the meaning of this?	How much?
	What is the nature of this?	How often?
		How big?
Typical methods	Interviews	Surveys
	Participant observation	
Explanatory/association		
Typical questions	What is happening here?	Does variable x
	What patterns exist?	relate to other
	How do phenomena differ and	variables?
	relate to each other?	What are the
		measurable
		associations between
		phenomena?
Typical methods	Observation	Cohort studies,
	Content analysis	surveys
		Quantitative
		statistical analysis
Hypothesis testing		
Typical questions	What difference does this	Is x more effective
	intervention make?	than y?
Typical methods	Survey/evaluation	Randomised
	Interview	controlled trial

(adapted from Miller & Crabtree 1992)

showed more uncertainty than low referrers, were less patient centred, and differed in other factors affecting referral decisions (Bailey *et al.* 1994).

Like many topics in primary care, variation in referral behaviour remains tantalisingly resistant to explanation and change. Even fundholding, which was supposed to give general practitioners an incentive to reduce referral rates did not do so (Surender *et al.* 1995). This body of research also has a subtext about the status and competence of general practice as compared to hospital medicine. For instance it is often assumed that the appropriateness of referrals to hospitals should be measured against standards set by hospital doctors. This subtext finds its way into research questions like 'do good doctors refer more patients to hospital?' (Reynolds *et al.* 1991); or a study of open access gastroscopy which starts by pointing out specialist unit concerns that the referral threshold might be lowered by open access (Hungin 1987).

Over the years a substantial body of general practice and primary care research has been published – a MEDLINE search from 1966 to the present on 'family practice/or general practice.tw or primary care.tw' yields 41 865 references. Marinker (1997) categorises several distinctive approaches to general practice – 'the illness as patient, as family, as risk, as community and as commodity', each of which is reflected in published research. The literature of general practice and primary care has expanded exponentially, with textbooks written from a primary care perspective by primary care doctors and nurses (for example the Oxford general practice series). The Royal College of General Practitioners has kept up a steady stream of occasional papers and other publications, and supports research in general practice through research training fellowships and grants.

The first academic department of general practice was established in Edinburgh in 1957 and the first chair, also in Edinburgh, in 1963 (Howie *et al.* 1986). However, there are still only 36 professors of general practice or primary care in the UK, and 400 posts in general practice in universities in England and Wales out of a total of 7343 medical academic posts. In 1997 there were 18 600 hospital consultants and 27 100 unrestricted general practice principals in England (Department of Health 1998a and 1998b). In 1995 there was one paid academic post per 124 GP principals in England and Wales, compared to 36 paid academic posts per 100 consultants (Royal College of General Practitioners 1997). However, the number of research papers written by service (non-academic) general practitioners is tiny. The proportion of original papers in the *British Journal of General Practice* written by service GPs fell from a half to a third in the 1980s (Pitts 1991), and by the first half of 1994 the proportion was 15% (Lipman 1996). The figures quoted above may even understate the true situation, as most publications from service GPs have come from a small group of enthusiasts.

This lack of service GP involvement in research is a serious barrier to the development of primary care as an academically based discipline whose practice is based on the findings of research. Although there are opportunities for (and encouragement to do) research during vocational training, the majority of full-time GPs have no protected time to do research (Pereira Gray 1991). The great silent majority of GPs has little interest in research and, especially over the last few years, has been struggling to meet increasing patient and administrative demands, leaving little time for academic pursuits. The very success of university departments of primary care, with ever-increasing sophistication in research methodology, and the (self-) selection of a small cohort of the most promising GP registrars to pursue an academic career immediately after completing vocational training, carries the danger of an élite group emerging which is perceived not to share the professional and financial preoccupations (and burdens) of most of the profession. In addition, GP researchers often meet with resentment and even hostility from their partners which occasionally leads to them either having to leave the partnership or curtail their research activities in order to meet their fair share of the workload. While it is plainly absurd to expect every GP to produce important research findings, health care routinely requires the *use* of research findings. Lack of experience in conducting research inevitably deprives many GPs of background knowledge and insight which could help them to make judgements about the validity, applicability and usefulness of the information with which they are daily bombarded by pharmaceutical companies, the medical and lay press, local advisors, consultant colleagues and many others.

During the last few years, initiatives such as the setting up of primary care research networks have been aimed at addressing some of these problems. There are now more than 20 of these throughout the country, with memberships ranging from under 20 to over 200 (Evans *et al.* 1997). The 1996 White Paper committed the government to establishing at least one primary care research network in each region by 1998 (Secretary of State for Health 1996). The networks vary in their organisation: some, such as the Yorkshire Primary Care Research Network (YReN, established in 1996), are organised by university departments of general practice; others, such as the Northern Primary Care Research Network (NoReN, established in 1992), are run by service GPs. NoReN runs a successful educational programme, offers support to individual practitioners in developing research projects, and organises larger scale projects involving several practices (see Boxes 3.3 and 3.4). It has also been successful in encouraging primary health care team members other than GPs to become involved in research.

Box 3.3: NoReN – the Northern Primary Care Research Network

History:	Established 1992 as an initiative by the Royal College of General Practitioners and the Northern Region NHSE
Background of lead coordinator (medical director):	General practice
Steering Committee:	Includes local academic representation, academic nurses, and general practitioners
Staff:	Medical director employed on a sessional basis and part-time secretary and research coordinator/facilitator
Membership:	Over 200 including practice nurses, health visitors and other non-medical primary care staff
Main activities:	Organising research training events (see Box 3.4), facilitating research practices, funding research fellows, organising multipractice research.

Guiding principles:
(1) Investing in people. Recognising that meaningful change is effected by motivated individuals and not by systems alone.

Contd

Box 3.3 *Contd*

(2)   Creating an environment in which research is seen as a positive attribute, part of everyday work and a necessity for the development of the individual and the profession.

(3)   Preparing a structured support system for fostering research by: (a) identifying areas of research; (b) providing planning advice; (c) technical and methodological assistance; (d) facilitating funding.

(4)   Developing an education and career structure for practice-based researchers including attachments and appointments to academic units, and to help people work towards higher degrees and diplomas in research.

(5)   Being part of an integrated drive towards research and development in primary health care and to ensure representation for primary care researchers at policy-making and resource allocation level.

Aims and objectives:

(1)   Training and education in research.

(2)   Supporting individual researchers and innovative research projects involving using both social science and biomedical methods.

(3)   Creating links between service general practitioners (practice-based researchers), the University, the RHA, the FHSAs, the RCGP and other bodies concerned with research in primary care.

(4)   Involving the entire primary health team in research.

(5)   Providing networking facilities to researchers: technical expertise, information technology, design and statistical planning, publication and information dissemination.

(6)   Assistance with research funding and practical help with funding applications.

(7)   Peer support and critical appraisal of projects.

(8)   Linking with a regional stratagem for research and development, including undergraduate and continuing medical education.

(9)   Linking with the international community of primary care researchers.

(10) Providing a forum for nationally and regionally decided research topics.

(11) Providing representation for practice-based researchers at policy-making and funding groups.

NoReN 1996

New methods of allocating research funding open up (at least in theory) opportunities for more research to be carried out by primary care (Carter 1997). The need for (and persisting lack of) a research culture in primary care has been recognised for many years; in particular, there is a need for research questions to emerge from within the clinical context of general practice rather than be imposed and investigated from without (O'Dowd 1995). It remains to be seen whether initiatives such as funding research general practices (in which one or more general practitioners in a practice are given funds to support research activities) will begin to reverse the

Box 3.4: NoReN activities 1995–96

May 1995	National Meeting on Primary Care Research Networks (31 participants)
June/July 1995	A short course in medical statistics (5 evening sessions, 7 participants)
July 1995	An introduction to research (basic training, 31 participants)
September 1995	Prescribing: challenges facing researchers in primary care and at the interface (26 participants)
September 1995	Diabetes: research priorities (26 participants)
November 1995	Annual research presentation day (121 participants – 51 papers presented; NoReN's policy is to encourage novice researchers to present work and the range varies from first attempts at research to work by experienced researchers awaiting peer review and publication)
January 1996	Research issues in the management of asthma in primary care (12 participants)
February 1996	Women's health research for primary care (17 participants)
February 1996	Clinical research in cardiovascular disease (11 participants)
March 1996	Counselling in primary care (37 participants)
March 1996	Gastroenterology: physical and functional aspects (8 participants)
March 1996	Exploring qualitative research in primary care (57 participants – a national meeting whose proceedings were later published as a supplement in *Family Practice* (Dec. 1996))
Special interest groups:	Prescribing Group, Women's Health Group, Cardiovascular Group, Cardiovascular Research Group, Diabetes Research Group, Gastroenterology Research Group. These groups meet several times a year and may hear presentations of research by members or outside speakers, discuss the early formulation of research questions, organise collaborative projects and give mutual support
Research development workshops:	Six informal meetings at members' surgeries or homes for peer support and advice on research projects

Training day for vocational trainers.

NoReN 1996

NHS research system's '[hostility] to general practice since 1948' (Pereira Gray 1995).

That said, research is not a high priority for most general practitioners, nor for the other, increasingly numerous, members of the primary health care team. Many consider it an achievement simply to cope with an incessant daily round of apparently ever-increasing patient demand. There has been an expansion in the range of services provided to patients which usually include well baby clinics, antenatal clinics and minor surgery, but may extend to asthma clinics, diabetes clinics, counselling, physiotherapy, dietetic advice and much else. A GP or primary care nurse might well declare 'We've got our hands full coping with looking after patients. We haven't got time to think about research. Anyway, what use is it to us?' Enthusiasts for research might respond 'To care for patients effectively, it is essential that clinicians understand and use the findings of research in their practice'. The remainder of this chapter is about how the need to implement findings of research has been approached in primary care, and about the impact upon and potential role of evidence-based practice in primary care.

The emergence and development of evidence-based practice in primary care

When evidence-based practice is mentioned, many clinicians retort, rather grumpily, that they have been using evidence in their practice for years. There is some justice in this response. The literature of general practice reflects a serious and sustained effort over several decades to examine and implement what is needed for high-quality primary care, both by carrying out research in the primary care setting, and by promoting and evaluating methods of achieving good practice. Much of this work has addressed issues that would later become part of the philosophy and methodology of evidence-based practice (see Box 3.5).

The importance of education in general practice (particularly in vocational training schemes) has long been recognised, and addressed

---

Box 3.5: Definition of evidence-based medicine* (Sackett *et al.* 1997)

'The practice of EBM is a process of life-long, self-directed learning in which caring for our own patients creates the need for clinically important information about diagnosis, prognosis, therapy and other clinical and health care issues, and in which we:

(1) convert these information needs into answerable questions;
(2) track down, with maximum efficiency, the best evidence with which to answer them (whether from the clinical examination, the diagnostic laboratory, from research evidence or other sources);
(3) critically appraise that evidence for its validity (closeness to the truth) and usefulness (clinical applicability);
(4) apply the results of this appraisal in our clinical practice; and
(5) evaluate our performance'.

*Although this definition refers to evidence-based medicine it plainly applies to any and all disciplines which use its principles, including nursing, purchasing, dentistry, midwifery and so on.

systematically (Royal College of General Practitioners 1972). Evidence-based practice is itself primarily an educational process, and there are many similarities with the approach taken by educators in general practice. Small-group learning has become a central part of the educational process in vocational training for general practice, for example (Greenhalgh 1997a). Perhaps the most important single skill which must be mastered for evidence-based practice is question forming, and this too is well recognised in general practice education (Fabb 1981).

Baker (1990) advocated clinical audit as a method for problem-solving and gave examples of successful and unsuccessful audits. This was analogous to the approach taken in evidence-based practice. Clinical audit emerged as an important tool for improving the quality of general practice in the early 1980s (Sheldon 1981). It equates to the evaluation stage in evidence-based practice and classically is envisaged as an audit cycle with four stages: set standards; measure current performance; compare practice with standards; and identify and remedy deviations from the standard. Then the cycle should be repeated to find out whether performance has improved (see Fig. 3.1).

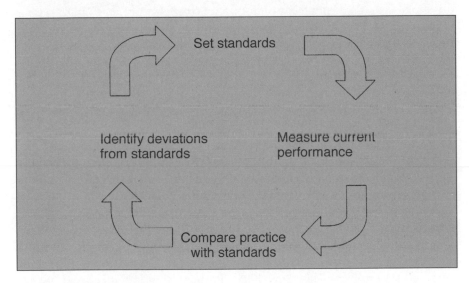

Fig. 3.1 The audit cycle.

When combined with ideas from the business world such as quality assurance and management, audit seemed to offer a way forward to improve the quality of care in general practice (Irvine 1990). This was in keeping with the *zeitgeist* of the Thatcher era, in which business methodology, as well as the inherent virtues of the market, was supposed to be applicable to and beneficial for all human activities.

The Royal College of General Practitioners launched its quality of care initiative in 1983 (Irvine 1983), with two aims, the second of which implicitly referred to audit (Buckley 1983) (see Box 3.6). 'Quality in Practice' bulletins were henceforth issued in the *Journal of the Royal College of General Practitioners*. These consisted of reports from the faculties and individual members of audits, study meetings, responsible prescribing and other quality issues. The bulletins make nostalgic reading now: plain, no-nonsense typed sheets, they display an earnest high-mindedness, a belief in good intentions, self-improvement and honest endeavour which, little more than a decade later, appears to belong to another age (see Box 3.6).

Box 3.6: Aims of the Royal College of General Practitioners' Quality of Care Initiative: adopted at a meeting of the College Council in June 1983

(1) Each general practitioner should describe his current work and be able to say what services he provides for his patients.
(2) Each general practitioner should define specific objectives for the care of his patients and should monitor the extent to which these objectives are met.

'As a first step in implementing these aims, each member of Council agreed to review aspects of his or her own practice and report back to Council' (Buckley 1983). Members of the regional Faculty Boards of the College were also expected to give a lead in implementing the quality initiative.

Medical audit advisory groups (MAAGs) were set up in 1990 'to direct, co-ordinate and monitor medical audit within all practices in their area' (Department of Health 1990). They have established a structure and process which enables primary care clinicians to examine critically the quality of care provided to patients (Spencer 1993). They have been careful to work by consensus and avoid antagonising potentially recalcitrant doctors. Many have employed lay staff to collect data for audits in order to reduce extra workload on the practice (Griew & Mortlock 1993). Most groups have comprised interested local GPs, although it was soon recognised that other members of the primary health care team such as nurses should be involved (Humphrey & Berrow 1993). Participation has increased, as has the quality of the audits, and multipractice audits have enabled MAAGs to tackle the problem of variation in practice by applying common standards across their area (Baker *et al.* 1995) (see Box 3.7).

During this period, opinion leaders in general practice began to tackle the problem of 'unacceptable delays in the implementation of many findings of research' (Haines & Jones 1994). There are many examples of these; one of the best known is the 13-year delay between the availability of evidence from meta-analysis of randomised controlled trials of the effec-

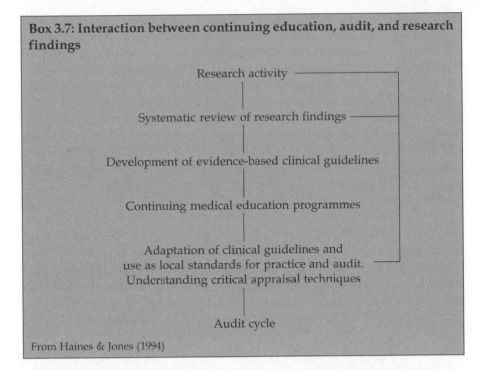

Box 3.7: Interaction between continuing education, audit, and research findings

Research activity

Systematic review of research findings

Development of evidence-based clinical guidelines

Continuing medical education programmes

Adaptation of clinical guidelines and use as local standards for practice and audit. Understanding critical appraisal techniques

Audit cycle

From Haines & Jones (1994)

tiveness of thrombolysis for myocardial infarction and the widespread acceptance (especially in medical textbooks) of the treatment (Antman *et al.* 1992). Haines and Jones (1994) recommend an integrated system, using a number of mechanisms, including education and audit, and acknowledging the need for understanding of critical appraisal techniques (see Box 3.7). This integrated system uses the established mechanisms of audit to set standards based upon evidence of clinical effectiveness. The evidence comes from evidence-based guidelines (Box 3.8), which are used as the source from which to set standards. Haines and Jones (1994) write of the need to 'implement research findings', in other words the process starts with the evidence, rather than individual patients' problems as in evidence-based practice (see back Box 3.5).

Knottnerus and Dinant (1997) point out the difficulties which clinicians have in using evidence from research which (in order to satisfy rigorous methodological criteria and demonstrate scientific validity) does not reflect the clinical problems they encounter in daily practice. They make a plea for researchers to provide 'medicine-based evidence' as an essential prerequisite for 'evidence-based medicine'. This is perhaps the central dilemma for any clinician seeking to base management of patients' problems on scientific evidence. Certainly it is a common complaint that the very patients whose complex problems are most in need of sound evidence with which to inform management are those who would not have fulfilled the inclusion criteria for the most rigorous and methodologically sound studies. A sceptic might observe that this demonstrates the inapplicability of evidence-based practice to routine clinical work. An enthusiast might respond that evidence-based practice, by raising important unanswered clinical questions, puts pressure on researchers to develop new methodologies to answer them.

> **Box 3.8: Evidence-based guidelines and consensus guidelines**
>
> Clinical guidelines have been defined as 'systematically developed statements to assist practitioner and patient decisions about appropriate health care for specific clinical circumstances' (Institute of Health 1992). Evidence-based guidelines are also systematic reviews of the literature, which use explicit methodology to ensure a thorough search for evidence, set explicit criteria for critically appraising it, and link recommendations and their strength to the evidence, and to its validity (Eccles *et al.* 1996). The user of evidence-based guidelines should be able to see whether the search for evidence was thorough and systematic, where the evidence has come from for each recommendation and why the recommendation has been made. Evidence-based guidelines should not be confused with less rigorously constructed consensus guidelines, disseminated by various expert groups over the years, which do not systematically review the literature, nor set explicit criteria for appraising evidence. Consensus guidelines' recommendations may not be reliable, as the user cannot assess the completeness or validity of evidence used to support them (Fink *et al.* 1984).

Projects to disseminate evidence-based practice in primary care have used the evidence-based guidelines and audit model as a vehicle both to increase the use of clinically effective interventions and to raise awareness of evidence-based practice. For example, the NEBPINY (Network for Evidence-Based Practice in Northern and Yorkshire) project introduced GPs and primary care nurses to the idea of asking questions about the care they were providing and gave them an opportunity to attend a critical appraisal workshop. Evidence-based guidelines were then introduced to the practices in order to select an intervention to set as a standard for a clinical audit. The Kings Fund PACE (Promoting Action on Clinical Effectiveness) programme, starting in 1996, has run 16 local projects across primary and secondary care, each concentrating on a single clinical problem (see Box 3.9). These single-topic projects are seen as a first step in learning about and encouraging evidence-based practice in a wider clinical context (Dunning *et al.* 1997).

The FACTS (Framework for Appropriate Care Throughout Sheffield) project has been running the Triple A programme since 1994 (Eve *et al.* 1997). The three As are: aspirin in secondary prevention of myocardial infarction and stroke; anti-coagulation in atrial fibrillation; and ACE inhi-

> **Box 3.9: The 16 local PACE projects**
>
> (1)   Barnet Health Authority – Hypertension
> (2)   Bradford Health Authority – *Helicobacter pylori* eradication
> (3)   Bromley – *Helicobacter pylori* eradication
> (4)   Chase Farm Hospital NHS Trust – Pressure sores
> (5)   Dorset Health Authority – Menorrhagia
> (6)   Dudley Health Authority – Continence
> (7)   Gloucestershire Royal NHS Trust – The management of stroke patients
> (8)   Lambeth, Southwark and Lewisham Health Authority and King's Health Care – Cardiac rehabilitation
> (9)   North Derbyshire Health Authority – Congestive cardiac failure
> (10) Oxfordshire Health Authority – Post-operative pain control
> (11) Royal Berkshire and Battle Hospitals NHS Trust – Leg ulcers
> (12) South Tyneside Health Care Trust – Stable angina
> (13) Southern Derbyshire – Low back pain
> (14) Walsall Health Authority – *Helicobacter pylori* eradication
> (15) Wigan and Bolton Health Authority – Continence
> (16) Wirral Health Authority – Family support in schizophrenia
>
> Dunning *et al.* 1997

bitors in heart failure. The project has considered very carefully how change in professional behaviour may be achieved and why so-called rational models (such as the dissemination of evidence-based guidelines) may not be taken up and used by clinicians. Much of the work has been qualitative and has sought to understand and bridge the cultural and conceptual gaps between the worlds of research, management, and everyday clinical practice.

These projects do not fulfil the criteria of evidence-based medicine as described in the work of David Sackett and his colleagues (Sackett *et al.* 1997). They set out in detail how clinicians could apply the principles of clinical epidemiology to the management of patients, and how, by learning to ask structured answerable questions, to search for information (evidence), and to critically appraise that evidence, they could both improve their clinical performance and keep up to date. The method is fundamentally educational and motivated by the clinician's questioning response to patients' problems (see Box 3.10). Unlike the guidelines/audit model, it requires clinicians not only to carry out certain tasks, but also to learn new skills (such as critical appraisal) and attitudes (such as how to recognise and act upon a gap in the clinician's own knowledge).

The response to evidence-based practice

Ridsdale (1996) correctly interprets evidence-based practice as primarily a learning process and advocates, whilst recognising the barrier of perfor-

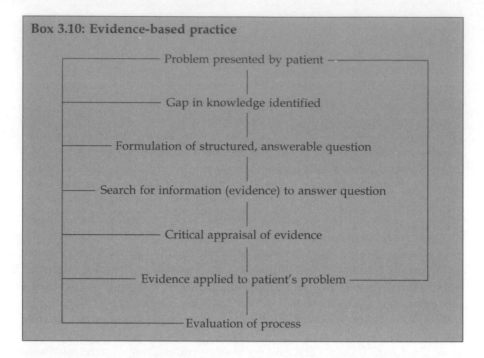

Box 3.10: Evidence-based practice

Problem presented by patient

Gap in knowledge identified

Formulation of structured, answerable question

Search for information (evidence) to answer question

Critical appraisal of evidence

Evidence applied to patient's problem

Evaluation of process

mance anxiety, that education in general practice should include database searching and critical appraisal skills. Dawes (1996) points out that searchable databases on CD-ROM such as the Cochrane Database of Systematic Reviews and the ACP Journal Club on Disc (now available as *Best Evidence* and including the journal *Evidence-Based Medicine*) contain a wealth of critically appraised material, and suggests that 'the practitioner who can find one hour a week in which to search and read will make huge strides'.

General practitioners and primary care nurses now regularly attend workshops on critical appraisal run by CASP (Critical Appraisal Skills Programme), which is based in Oxford but has run workshops throughout the UK. These cascading workshops were designed to encourage others to run their own workshops (Centre for Evidence-Based Medicine 1997). For example, workshops are now being run in the North-East of England by CANNY (Critical Appraisal in Northern and Yorkshire), and there are also individual initiatives such as an evidence-based journal club for primary care nurses (Karen Jones, personal communication).

Following David Sackett's move to Oxford in 1994, the NHS Reviews and Dissemination Centre for Evidence-Based Medicine (CEBM) was opened at the John Radcliffe Hospital in March 1995. Five-day UK workshops on teaching evidence-based medicine have been held annually since then at Oxford and in London, and there have also been workshops in Cardiff, in addition to shorter workshops, such as the three-day 'How to practice evidence-based child health' workshops at the Centre for Evidence-Based Child Health in London. All of these attract general practitioners and primary care nurses, both as participants and as tutors. A number of general practitioners are members of the Centre and have, with others, been active in the organisation of evidence-based medicine workshops, taking the lead in Cardiff and London, for example.

However, Greenhalgh (1997b) asks 'why do people often groan when you mention evidence-based medicine?' and points out the 'palpable resentment among many health professionals towards the evidence-based medicine movement'. Primary care clinicians have to cope with an unending pressure of demand from patients, they may already have undergone extensive postgraduate or other professional training, and regularly attend postgraduate educational events in a conscientious attempt to keep up to date. The implications that their educational activities are ineffective, that they are not, after all, up to date and that they should now turn their established attitudes and behaviour upside down, are threatening, and may be perceived as insulting. They must learn new skills such as database searching and critical appraisal, and become familiar with technical terms and concepts such as absolute risk, relative risk, number needed to treat, likelihood ratio and so on. Experienced health professionals who decide to learn how to apply evidence-based practice implicitly accept the almost forgotten role of student, or novice. It would be surprising if they were entirely comfortable with this.

Misunderstandings as to the nature of evidence-based practice often distort discussion about it. The false assumption that evidence-based practice is concerned mainly or only with randomised controlled trials as applied to clearly defined diseases, or that it 'can only be conducted from ivory towers and armchairs' is widespread despite rebuttals from its leading advocates (Sackett *et al.* 1996). A common misconception is that evidence-based practice over-emphasises 'a simple biomedical approach or the use of randomised controlled trials' or ignores 'concerns about the applicability of the available biomedical evidence to general practice' (Jacobsen *et al.* 1997). Sweeney (1996) worries that 'EBM measures only what is measurable', and assumes that it has no part to play where 'problems are not exclusively biomedical, but reflect personal, social or cultural issues'. There is a philosophical and even ideological reaction against evidence-based practice by those concerned primarily to maintain and foster a holistic approach to patient care, which is sometimes vehement to the point of outright hostility. Sowerby (1977) elegantly anticipated and refuted these arguments by pointing out that Balint's psychoanalytic approach often led participants in Balint groups to ignore clinical diagnoses (indeed to presuppose that psychological factors were more important), and advocated that general practice must 'return to a primarily scientific orientation'. Unfortunately many arguments used against evidence-based practice are based on caricature rather than fact, and are unhelpful in addressing the very real problems of its application in daily general practice. For example, it would be perfectly reasonable to observe that the description of 'integrating individual clinical expertise with the best available external clinical evidence' in the textbook by Sackett *et al.* (1997) gives little detailed guidance on exactly how to do it, but unreasonable to assert that it cannot (and some would say should not) be done at all.

Many people (including clinicians, but especially managers) assume too that, wherever evidence of clinical effectiveness is put into practice (as in guidelines and audit projects), then evidence-based practice is taking place. Others think that evidence-based medicine is plainly impracticable in a clinical setting where only five to ten minutes is allowed for each patient contact: sceptics tend to ask whether it is necessary or feasible to do a MEDLINE search at each consultation. There is also an unfortunate tendency for some clinicians to claim that their practice is evidence-based by citing the findings of research to support their practice without having critically appraised the evidence in any meaningful way.

A questionnaire survey of GPs' perceptions about evidence-based medicine (McColl *et al.* 1998) found that the majority broadly welcomed the idea of evidence-based medicine, thought that it improved patient care and agreed that research findings were useful in the day-to-day management of patients. However, they believed that their colleagues were less welcoming and perceived organisational and personal inertia, patients' expectations, and lack of hard evidence to be barriers to evidence-based practice. They had a low level of awareness of databases and review publications such as *Bandolier*, *Effective Health Care Bulletins*, *Cochrane Library* or the journal *Evidence-Based Medicine*, and few had used any of these to help in clinical decision-making. Only 5% of respondents believed that learning the skills of evidence-based medicine was the most appropriate method of moving forward from 'opinion-based medicine', while 37% favoured seeking and applying evidence-based summaries, and 57% favoured evidence-based guidelines or protocols (McColl *et al.* 1998).

The relevance of evidence-based practice for primary care

The notion of self-directed learning contradicts the long-established traditions of medical and nursing education – i.e. that there is a body of knowledge, 'owned' by experts, who are the only people competent both to decide what that body of knowledge is and to teach it. GPs are often much more comfortable with this model than with the subversive, apparently anarchic, evidence-based process and this is reflected in the findings of studies such as that of McColl *et al.* (1998). The audit process is familiar to primary health care teams and is being widely used as the route to evidence-based practice (Eve *et al.* 1997; Dunning *et al.* 1997). However, single projects (or even several projects in a locality) only provide evidence to inform a small proportion of the GPs' workload. For example, a project to implement five evidence-based guidelines in Newcastle and North Tyneside would have influenced fewer than 3% of GPs' consultations (Lipman 1998a). The logistical problems of implementing evidence-based guidelines for most of the primary care workload would be formidable.

A small minority of GPs are enthusiastic about the potential of evidence-based practice for primary care. Its skills are seen as empowering the GP, not only to keep up to date more effectively, but also to 'educate, defend and negotiate on behalf of patients in a true primary care led National Health Service' (Rogers 1997). A group of GPs, reflecting on their experiences at the third UK workshop on teaching evidence-based medicine, identified ten characteristics and effects which they thought would apply to evidence-based practice in primary care (Lipman *et al.* 1997) (see Box 3.11).

Box 3.11: Characteristics and effects of evidence-based practice in primary care

(1) Empowering the primary care doctor
(2) Enabling the role as patient's advocate
(3) Informing the role of purchaser and commissioner of health care
(4) Effective and informed gatekeeping
(5) Easy access to evidence*
(6) Encouraging improvement of skills and education
(7) Improved professional development
(8) Keeping up to date with literature
(9) Rekindling curiosity
(10) Regarding evidence-based medicine as a tool and not a panacea
     (discussion held on 11 July 1996)

*a necessary condition for evidence-based practice

Lipman *et al.* 1997

It is important to recognise that the 'empowerment' of GPs practising evidence-based medicine could imply a relative disempowerment of other clinicians such as nurses. Greenhalgh and Douglas (1998) found that nurses and doctors in primary care had different perceptions of what research and evidence meant. Doctors were more likely to express a narrow view, which most valued generalisable quantitative evidence (such as from clinical trials), whereas nurses included qualitative research, local information and even anecdote as research evidence. The confusion about terminology compounds a situation where many primary care clinicians (especially nurses) feel isolated and unsupported and risks leading to their initial suspicions about evidence-based practice growing into outright hostility and alienation. So, while evidence-based practice may have great potential to enhance primary care, there are many barriers to be overcome first.

Terminology is a barrier in two ways. First, evidence-based practice requires its practitioners to understand and use technical terms such as sensitivity, specificity, relative risk, absolute risk and so on, and understand the nature of different research methodologies. This adds clarity to the formulation of questions, aids the search for evidence, and is fundamental to critical appraisal. If done properly, it enables practitioners to extract the maximum information from evidence, but the techniques and technical terms must be learned, and they can be intimidating at first, as can initial experiences with database searching.

Second, the term evidence-based medicine implies that medicine, particularly specialist hospital medicine, is the dominant paradigm in evidence-based practice. If a doctor uses it carelessly in mixed company he or she will rightly be corrected, usually by a nurse, who will insist that it should be evidence-based *practice* (personal communication on many occasions from evidence-based nurses!). Therefore evidence-based practice, or evidence-based health care are now used as generic terms, with evidence-based nursing, evidence-based psychiatry and so on indicating that each professional group must find its own way to apply the principles originally described as 'evidence-based medicine'.

How does all this help the primary care clinician in practice? First, a practical understanding of clinical epidemiology can be extremely useful to the primary care clinician. As long ago as 1985 Knottnerus described the way prevalence of illness influences the predictive value of diagnostic signs, symptoms and tests in different clinical settings, in a manner which would not be out of place in a current text on evidence-based practice. He pointed out that these differences mean that general practitioners and specialists must adopt different diagnostic strategies and warned against transferring findings uncritically from one setting to another (Knottnerus 1985). GPs have always been aware that their patients are different from hospital patients – for example a headache presented in a GP's Monday morning surgery carries a much lower risk of signifying a brain tumour than it does in a neurology outpatient clinic.

Sackett *et al.* (1991) describe the properties of diagnostic tests (sensitivity, specificity, predictive values and likelihood ratios) and how to use them. For example the likelihood ratio for coronary artery stenosis (the ratio between the likelihood that patients with and without a positive diagnostic test, clinical sign or symptom will in reality have the target disease) of a classic history of angina of effort is far greater than that of a positive exercise ECG (electrocardiogram). This is extremely valuable information if the GP understands its significance. If a patient presents with rather vague chest pains, the history does not suggest angina, and is at low risk of developing angina in the first place, then an exercise ECG test is likely at best to be useless, and at worst harmful. If GPs are aware of this they will resist the temptation to order an exercise ECG just to be on the safe side. A negative result would merely confirm what is already most likely, but a positive test would not only not confirm angina but in most cases is much more likely to be a false positive test than a true positive. In other words, ordering the test has no potential for benefit but much potential for harm by unnecessarily raising patients' anxieties (see Box 3.12).

Box 3.12: True positive, false positive, true negative and false negative rates for exercise ECG as a diagnostic test for coronary artery stenosis at prevalence rates of 1%, 5%, 10% and 50%

Prevalence	True Positive	False Positive	True Negative	False Negative
1%	0.7%	11.9%	87.1%	0.3%
5%	3.4%	11.4%	83.6%	1.6%
10%	6.9%	10.8%	79.2%	3.1%
50%	34.5%	6%	44.0%	15.5%

These can be worked out in a few minutes using 2×2 tables if sensitivity and specificity are known for the test. In this case sensitivity = 69% and specificity = 88%.

Martin *et al.* 1992

Likelihood ratios can be used with a nomogram to generate post-test probabilities from pre-test probabilities derived from epidemiological evidence and clinical judgement (Fagan 1975). It is suggested that clinical biochemistry test reports should include likelihood ratios for the tests rather than normal ranges. In order to take full advantage of this, GPs will have to know how to use them in conjunction with the history and physical examination. For example, in biochemical testing for hypothyroidism, the pre-test probability in patients without a suggestive history is around 1% and a positive test gives a post-test probability of under 30%, but if the patient has several signs and symptoms of hypothyroidism, the post-test probability after a positive test is over 90% (Moore 1998).

The history and clinical examination have long been known to contribute more to the diagnosis than laboratory or other investigations (Hampton *et al.* 1975). Clinical epidemiology makes their interpretation more precise and more useful. Primary care clinicians use many strategies to make diagnoses, such as asking questions about general well-being ('Is he still eating?' 'Is she still drinking?'); timing of symptoms ('Did the headache start all of a sudden?' 'Is it worse in the morning?'); or other factors ('Is it worse when you bend down?' 'Is it better after food?'). This is potentially an exciting area of research in primary care, as these kinds of questions are really tests, and will have sensitivity, specificity and likelihood ratios for many illnesses. These could be measured by cohort studies in primary care and would transform the process of diagnosis.

The second area of potential benefit involves the self-directed educational process of evidence-based practice. There is evidence that a problem-based educational approach in undergraduates produces doctors who keep more up to date than those who have had traditional didactic teaching (Shin & Haynes 1991). It has also been shown that GPs' level of knowledge declines steadily throughout their careers after completing training (van Leeuwen *et al.* 1995). This is worrying at a time when the pace of developments in medicine is more rapid than ever before. Introducing self-directed learning based upon problems arising out of their own clinical practice is perhaps the most promising strategy both to remedy the trend towards declining knowledge among established general practitioners and to enable them to keep up to date with rapid and manifold changes in clinical knowledge and practice.

Fortunately the technology now exists to support evidence-based practice in primary care. Computers are widely used and it is simple to install databases such as the Cochrane Library on CD-ROM or *Best Evidence* (structured abstracts with critical appraisals of important and valid papers which have been published in the *ACP* (American College of Physicians) *Journal Club* or *Evidence-Based Medicine* journal). MEDLINE is available over the Internet and will soon be available, along with other databases such as Embase and CINAHL (the Cumulative Index of Nursing and Allied Health Literature), from the NHS network. Thus primary care clinicians can now access evidence in their own clinical settings without having to make time-consuming journeys to the local postgraduate centre.

Self-directed small group learning at their place of work would be the main educational activity for evidence-based primary care practitioners (although external courses and workshops would still have an important role). Responsibility for identifying and meeting educational needs would be devolved to clinicians. Primary care nurses in particular would be able to develop their professions in new ways. Changes in practice would be informed by the information they have gained in response to their patients' problems, rather than being imposed upon them by hierarchies, which may not necessarily share or understand their experience.

The third important consequence of evidence-based practice in primary care is the confidence it gives practitioners to make up their own minds about clinical matters, and not to rely on received authority. This will undoubtedly affect the relationship with secondary care, because primary care clinicians will jettison their long-established instinct of deference to specialists, and also because they will tend to make more precise referrals, in which clinical questions can be more clearly formulated than hitherto.

This ought to be helpful to consultants, although some might be irritated if they think their judgement or knowledge is being questioned. However, they might reflect that it will be a great advance on the kind of referral letter which used to request the consultant to 'please see and treat'! It should also banish the kind of absurdity exemplified by the 'right' answers in the MRCGP examination in the early 1980s being ascertained by 'the simple expedient of looking up the relevant specialist textbook' (Norell 1984).

The relationship between primary care and the pharmaceutical industry may also benefit from evidence-based practice. GPs will be able to understand whether or not promotional material is useful or accurate (for instance by understanding that a relative risk reduction needs to be translated to an absolute risk reduction to be clinically meaningful). The present situation, where attitudes vary between hair-shirted avoidance of anything to do with drug companies and thoughtless acceptance of any old data, provided it comes with a free meal and a postgraduate education allowance certificate, will change. The former attitude is as ridiculous as the latter, and patient care can only benefit if a meaningful dialogue, based on the ability to critically appraise evidence and examine important therapeutic questions, is established between the users and developers of therapies.

There is some unease and doubt about the value of an evidence-based approach within the consultation. This may be because there is a perception that individual patients' stories, which are the everyday subject of primary care, are relegated to a low position in the hierarchy of evidence. Randomised controlled trials, which 'produce an oversimplified and artificial environment which may bear little resemblance to day-to-day reality', are usually placed at the top (Sullivan & MacNaughton 1996). However, it is precisely because evidence such as from randomised controlled trials is difficult to relate to daily reality that clinicians must understand them and learn how to interpret them for the needs of their individual patients. In primary care many questions are not answerable by randomised controlled trials, but it would be a mistake to infer from this that evidence-based practice is only rarely possible. Sackett and Wennberg (1997) point out that different questions require different research designs and that arguing over which is the best is a waste of time. In the same way, structured answerable questions in primary care may lead the practitioner to qualitative research, cohort studies, descriptive studies and so on, which can be critically appraised and used to answer the questions.

In the consultation itself, an evidence-based approach starts initially with the formulation of questions. These questions can be shared with patients so that they understand their problems and the options open to them better and can share in decision-making. This makes the clinician both student and teacher – remember the etymology of the word 'doctor' coming from the Latin *docere*, to teach or lead out. For example, the patient can be drawn into the decision-making process by formulating the problem as a question, 'What might you gain by treating your high blood pressure?' and answering it by demonstrating their risk of cardiovascular disease and how it can be reduced (Lipman 1998b).

What is the significance of evidence-based practice in primary care?

Evidence-based practice is not simply about evaluating and implementing the findings of research. It is essentially an educational process, which takes as its starting point the problems brought to clinicians by patients. In primary care this means that, for the first time, individual clinicians and primary health care teams can, if they wish, identify the knowledge they need to inform their clinical practice directly according to their patients' needs. The inevitable discovery of gaps in the availability of evidence to answer their questions will stimulate the formulation of research questions relevant to their practice.

The permission which evidence-based practice gives not only to admit ignorance without censure, but to use it to identify and learn what we need to know, is a radical change in the culture of clinicians, both frightening (at first!) and liberating. It is no respecter of hierarchy or autocracy. GPs may welcome it when they discover that it increases their professional autonomy, but they will also have to accept that it will do the same for nurses and other clinicians.

Evidence-based practice will transform continuing professional education, which will become integrated into the daily clinical routine. Developments in information technology will make the finding of evidence straightforward, and enable it to be incorporated into the patient's record. Websites with evidence-based information could encourage the use of self-directed learning and self-care among patients themselves. Purves (1996) describes the use of computers for decision and knowledge support, virtual encounters (in which patient and clinician interact asynchronously with the computer), and computer support for patient-focused self-learning.

The consequences of not acquiring the skills of evidence-based practice would include: increasing difficulty for clinicians in keeping up to date; overreliance on bureaucratic processes to achieve a limited number of clinically effective interventions; and gradual erosion of professional autonomy. Perhaps most important would be the loss of the opportunity to combine an individual patient-centred approach to health care with the use of the most effective interventions.

The skills of evidence-based practice should be seen as complementing the existing skills of primary care rather than replacing them. However, they have the potential to transform the way primary care goes about its tasks and to irrevocably change attitudes towards diagnosis and treatment. A firm grasp of how to interpret evidence and integrate it into the care of individual patients is likely to exert strong pressure on practitioners to avoid procedures they know to be ineffective. It will be increasingly difficult for clinicians to invoke the mantra of clinical freedom when doing something plainly at odds with the evidence, such as prescribing antibiotics for the common cold. This will change relationships with patients – and may cause initial tensions as clinicians have to explain why they can no longer agree to prescribe a treatment which patients have come to expect. Ultimately, however, the evidence-based process, in which the questions asked by and choices available to patients and clinicians are made explicit, will lead both to improved clinical effectiveness, and to a more open, honest and productive partnership between patient and clinician.

References

Antman E., Lau J., Kupeltruck B., Mosteller F. & Chalmers I. (1992) A comparison of the results of meta-analyses of randomised controlled trials and recommendations of clinical experts. *Journal of the American Medical Association*, **268**, 240–48.

Bailey J., King N. & Newton P. (1994) Analysing general practitioners' referral decisions II. Applying the analytical framework: do high and low referrers differ in factors influencing their referral decisions? *Family Practice*, **11**, 9–14.

Baker R. (1990) Problem solving with audit in general practice. *British Medical Journal*, **300**, 378–80.

Baker R., Hearnshaw H., Cooper A., Cheater F. & Robertson N. (1995) Assessing the work of medical audit advisory groups in promoting audit in general practice. *Quality in Health Care*, **4**, 234–9.

Balint M. (1964) *The Doctor, his Patient and the Illness*. Pitman, London.

Britten N., Jones R., Murphy E. & Stacy R. (1995) Qualitative research methods in general practice and primary care. *Family Practice*, **12**, 104–14.

Buckley E.G. (1983) Quality and the College. *Journal of the Royal College of General Practitioners*, **33**, 761.

Buckley G. (1995) Projects revisited. *Education for General Practice*, **6**, 79.

Byrne P.S. & Long B.E.L. (1976) *Doctors Talking to Patients*. HMSO, London.

Carter Y. (1997) Funding research in primary care: is Culyer the remedy? *British Journal of General Practice*, **47**, 544–5.

Coulter A. (1992) The interface between primary and secondary care. In M. Roland & A. Coulter (eds) *Hospital Referrals*. Oxford University Press, Oxford.

Coulter A., Seagroatt V. & McPherson K. (1990) Relation between general practices' outpatient referrral rates and rates of elective admission to hospital. *British Medical Journal*, **301**, 273–6.

Cummins R.O., Jarman B. & White P.M. (1981) Do general practitioners have different 'referral thresholds'? *British Medical Journal*, **282**, 1037–9.

Dawes M. (1996) On the need for evidence-based general and family practice. *Evidence-Based Medicine*, **1**, 68–9.

Department of Health (1990) *Medical Audit in the Family Practitioner Services.* HC(FP)(90)8, DoH, London.

Department of Health (1998a) *NHS General Medical Services: Unrestricted principals by contractual commitment at 1 October.*
http://www.doh.gov.uk/HPSSS/TBL_D6.HTM

Department of Health (1998b) *NHS Hospital and Community Health Services: Medical and dental staff at 30 September.* http://www.doh.gov.uk/HPSS/TBL_D2.HTM

Dunning M., Abl-Aad G., Gilbert D., Gillam S. & Livett H. (1997) *Turning Evidence into Everyday Practice.* King's Fund, London.

Eccles M., Clapp Z., Grimshaw J., Adams P.C., Higgins B., Purves I. & Russel I. (1996) North of England evidence-based guidelines development project: methods of guidelines development. *British Medical Journal*, **312**, 760–62.

Evans D., Exworthy M., Peckham S., Robinson R. & Day P. (1997) *Primary care research networks report.* NHS Executive South and West Research & Development Directorate.

Eve R., Golton I., Hodgkin P., Munro J. & Musson G. (1997) *Learning from FACTS: lessons from the Framework for Appropriate Care Throughout Sheffield project.* ScHARR Occasional paper no.97/3. School of Health and Related Research, University of Sheffield, Sheffield.

Fabb W.E. (1981) Continuing education – identifying our needs. *Journal of the Royal College of General Practitioners*, **31**, 395–400.

Fagan T.J. (1975) Nomogram for Bayes's Theorem. *New England Journal of Medicine*, **293**, 257.

Fairhurst K., May C. (1995) Consumerism and the consultation: the doctor's view. *Family Practice*, **12**, 389–91.

Fertig A., Roland M., King H. & Moore T.R. (1993) Understanding variation in rates of referral among general practitioners: are inappropriate referrals important and would guidelines help to reduce rates? *British Medical Journal*, **307**, 1467–70.

Fink A., Kosekoff J., Chassin M. & Brook R. (1984) Consensus methods: characteristics and guidelines for use. *American Journal of Public Health*, **74**, 979–83.

Fry J. (1959) Why patients go to hospital: a study of usage. *British Medical Journal*, **(i)**, 1322–7.

Greenhalgh P. & Douglas H.R. (1998) *'Life's too short and the evidence too hard to find': a training needs analysis of GPs and practice nurses in evidence based-practice in North Thames Region.* Unit for Evidence-Based Practice and Policy, Department of Primary Care and Population Sciences, University College London, London.

Greenhalgh T. (1997a) Workshops for teaching evidence-based practice. *Evidence-Based Medicine*, **3**, 7–8.

Greenhalgh T. (1997b) *How to Read a Paper: the Basics of Evidence-Based Medicine.* BMJ Publishing Group, London.

Griew K. & Mortlock M. (1993) A study of MAAG organisation and function. *Audit Trends*, **3**, 89–93.

Haines A. & Jones R. (1994) Implementing findings of research. *British Medical Journal*, **308**, 1488–92.

Hampton J.R., Harrison M.J.G., Mitchell J.R.A., Prichard J.S. & Seymour C. (1975) Relative contributions of history-taking, physical examination, and laboratory investigation to diagnosis and management of medical outpatients. *British Medical Journal*, **(ii)**, 486–9.

Hart J.T. (1974) The marriage of primary care and epidemiology: the Milroy lecture, 1974. *Journal of the Royal College of Physicians of London*, **8**, 299–314.

Heath I. (1995) *The Mystery of General Practice*. Nuffield Provincial Hospitals Trust, London.

Howie J.G.R., Hannay D.R. & Stevenson J.S.K. (1986) *The Mackenzie Report: General Practice in the Medical Schools of the United Kingdom*. Department of General Practice, University of Edinburgh, Edinburgh.

Humphrey C. & Berrow D. (1993) Developing role of medical audit advisory groups. *Quality in Health Care*, **2**, 232–8.

Hungin A.S. (1987) Use of an open-access gastroscopy service by a general practice: findings and subsequent specialist referrral rate. *Journal of the Royal College of General Practitioners*, **37**, 170–71.

Hutton W. (1995) *The State We're In*. Jonathan Cape, London.

Institute of Health (1992) *Guidelines for Clinical Practice: From Development to Use*, Field M.J. & Lohr K.N. (eds). National Academic Press, Washington DC.

Irvine D.H. (1983) Quality of care in general practice: our outstanding problem. *Journal of the Royal College of General Practitioners*, **33**, 521–3.

Irvine D.H. (1985) *Chairman's Report to the Spring General Meeting, Cambridge, March 1985*. Quality in Practice: a Bulletin from the Royal College of General Practitioners. Royal College of General Practitioners, London.

Irvine D.H. (1990) *Managing for Quality in General Practice*. King's Fund Centre for Health Services Development, London.

Jacobsen L.D., Edwards A.G.K., Granier S.K. & Butler C.C. (1997) Evidence-based medicine and general practice. *British Journal of General Practice*, **47**, 449–52.

Knottnerus J.A. (1985) Interpretation of diagnostic data: an unexplored field in general practice. *Journal of the Royal College of General Practitioners*, **35**, 270–74.

Knottnerus J.A. & Dinant G.J. (1997) Medicine-based evidence: a prerequisite for evidence-based medicine. *British Medical Journal*, **315**, 1109–10.

Knottnerus J.A., Joosten J. & Daams J. (1990) Comparing the quality of referrals of general practitioners with high and average referral rates: an independent panel review. *British Journal of General Practice*, **40**, 178–81.

Lipman T. (1996) GP research: publish or be damned? *Royal College of General Practitioners North of England Faculty Newsletter*, **22**, 2.

Lipman T. (1998a) Discrepancies exist between general practitioners' clinical work and a guidelines implementation programme [Letter]. *British Medical Journal*, **317**, 604.

Lipman T. (1998b) Homage to Kilgore Trout: towards the evidence-based consultation. *British Journal of General Practice*, **48**, 1028–9.

Lipman T., Rogers S. & Jones Elwyn G. (1997) Evidence-based medicine in general practice: some views from the 3rd UK workshop on teaching evidence-based medicine. *Evidence-Based Medicine*, **2**, 133–5.

Mackichan N. (1976) *The GP and the Primary Health Care Team*. Pitman, London.

Marinker M. (1997) General Practice and the Millenium. *RCGP Members Reference Book 1997/98*: 256–7.

Marsh G.N. (1991) *Efficient Care in General Practice*. Oxford University Press, Oxford.

Martin T.W., Seaforth J.F. & Johns J.P. (1992) Comparison of exercise electrocardiography and dopamine echocardiography. *Clinical Cardiology*, **15**, 641–6.

McColl A., Smith H., White P. & Field J. (1998) General practitioners perceptions of the route to evidence-based medicine: a questionnaire survey. *British Medical Journal*, **316**, 361–5.

Miller W.L. & Crabtree B.F. (eds) (1992) *Doing Qualitative Research*. Sage, London.

Moore R.A. (1998) On the need for evidence-based clinical biochemistry. *Evidence-Based Medicine*, **3**, 7–8.

Neighbour R. (1987) *The Inner Consultation: How to Develop an Effective and Intuitive Consultation Style*. Kluwer Academic Publishers, London.

NHS Executive (1996) *NHS Annual Report 1995/6*. NHS Executive, Leeds.

NHS Executive North Thames Region (1998) *Clinical Governance in North Thames: a paper for discussion and consultation*. NHSE North Thames Region Office, London.

NHS Review and Dissemination Centre for Evidence-Based Medicine (1997) *Status Report 1997*. Centre for Evidence-Based Medicine, Oxford.

Norell J.S. (1984) What every doctor knows. William Pickles lecture 1984. *Journal of the Royal College of General Practitioners*, **34**, 417–24.

Northern Primary Care Research Network (NoReN) (1996) *Report 1995–96*.

O'Dowd T. (1995) Research in general practice: who is calling the tune? *British Journal of General Practice*, **45**, 515.

Oswald N. (1992) The history and development of the referral system. In M. Roland & A. Coulter (eds) *Hospital Referrals*. Oxford University Press, Oxford.

Pendleton D., Schofield T., Tate P. & Havelock P. (1984) *The Consultation: an Approach to Learning and Teaching*. Oxford University Press, Oxford.

Pereira Gray D. (1991) Research in general practice: law of inverse opportunity. *British Medical Journal*, **302**, 1380–82.

Petchey R., Williams J. & Baker M. (1997) 'Ending up a GP': a qualitative study of junior doctors' perceptions of general practice as a career. *Family Practice*, **14**, 194–8.

Pickles W. (1939) *Epidemiology in a Country Practice*. John Wright, London. (Reprinted RCGP, London, 1984).

Pitts J. (1991) General practice research in the Journal. *British Journal of General Practice*, **41**, 34–5.

Purves I. (1996) Facing future challenges in general practice: a clinical method with computer support. *Family Practice*, **13**, 536–43.

Reynolds G.A., Chitnis J.G. & Roland M.O. (1991) General practitioner outpatient referrals: do good doctors refer more patients to hospital? *British Medical Journal*, **302**, 1250–52.

Ridsdale L. (1996) Evidence-based learning for general practice. *British Journal of General Practice*, **46**, 503–504.

Rogers S. (1997) Evidence-based learning for general practice [letter]. *British Journal of General Practice*, **47**, 52–3.

Rowsell R., Morgan M. & Sarangi J. (1995) General practitioner registrars' views about a career in general practice. *British Journal of General Practice*, **45**, 601–604.

Royal College of General Practitioners (1969) The educational needs of the future general practitioner. *Journal of the Royal College of General Practitioners*, **18**, 358–60.

Royal College of General Practitioners (1972) *The Future General Practitioner: Learning and Teaching*. Royal College of General Practitioners, London.

Royal College of General Practitioners (1992) *The European Study of Referrals from Primary to Secondary Care*. Occasional paper no. 56. Royal College of General Practitioners, London.

Royal College of General Practitioners (1997) *RCGP Members' Reference Book 1997/98*, xxv.

Sackett D.L., Haynes B.L., Guyatt G.H. & Tugwell P. (1991) *Clinical Epidemiology: a Basic Science for Clinical Medicine* (2nd edition). Little, Brown and Company, Boston.

Sackett D.L., Richardson W.S., Rosenberg W. & Haynes R.B. (1997) *Evidence-Based Medicine: How to Practice and Teach EBM*. Churchill Livingstone, London.

Sackett D.L., Rosenberg W.M.C., Gray J.A.M., Haynes R.B. & Richardson W.S. (1996) Evidence-based medicine: what it is and what it isn't. *British Medical Journal*, **312**, 71–2.

Sackett D.L. & Wennberg J.E. (1997) Choosing the best research design for each question: it's time to stop squabbling over the 'best' methods. *British Medical Journal*, **315**, 1636.

Secretary of State for Health (1996) *Primary Care: Delivering the Future*. Department of Health, London.

Secretary of State for Health (1997) *The New NHS: Modern, Dependable*. HMSO, London.

Sheldon M. (1981) *Medical Audit in General Practice*. Royal College of General Practitioners (Occasional Paper 20), London.

Shin J. & Haynes R.B. (1991) Does a problem-based, self-directed undergraduate medical curriculum promote continuing clinical competence? *Clinical Research*, **39**, 143A.

Sowerby P. (1977) Balint Reassessed. The doctor, his patient and the illness: a reappraisal. *Journal of the Royal College of General Practitioners*, **27**, 583–9.

Spencer J. (1993) Audit in general practice: where do we go from here? *Quality in Health Care*, **2**, 183–8.

Sullivan F.M. & MacNaughton R.J. (1996) Evidence in consultations: interpreted and individualised. *Lancet*, **348**, 941–3.

Surender R., Bradlow J., Coulter A., Doll H. & Stewart Brown S. (1995) Prospective study of trends in referral patterns in fundholding and non-fundholding practices in the Oxford region, 1990–94. *British Medical Journal*, **311**, 1205–8.

Sweeney K. (1996) How can evidence-based medicine help patients in general practice? *Family Practice*, **13**, 498–90.

Swift G. (1982) Recollections and reflections: general practice since 1946, the George Swift Lecture. *Journal of the Royal College of General Practitioners*, **32**, 471–9.

van Leewen Y.D., Mol S.S.L., Pollemans M.C., Drop M.J., Grol R. & van der Vleuten C.P.M. (1995) Change in knowledge of general practitioners during their professional careers. *Family Practice*, **12**, 313–17.

Widgery D. (1991) *Some Lives: a GP's East End*. Sinclair-Stevenson, London.

Chapter 4

Evidence-Based Practice in Mental Health

John Geddes

Introduction

Evidence-based practice has had a particular impact in mental health. As well described by Parry (1992) (writing about psychotherapy), one of the main forces for change has been the demand of consumers and third-party payers in the 1980s and 1990s for evidence of the comparative effectiveness and costs of both psychological and pharmacological treatments. These pressures have forced the various disciplines in mental health services (e.g. clinical psychology, psychiatry, mental health nursing) to begin to work together, providing evidence for the effectiveness of their treatments. Although this has been a somewhat painful process, there are signs that it has made practitioners begin to appreciate the importance of evidence, and made researchers appreciate the importance of making research clinically applicable. The rise of managed care in the US in the 1980s sharpened this debate but also made it essential for different disciplines to try to speak the same language of research; and also to begin to base their clinical practice on evidence.

In this chapter I will review the implications and current development of evidence-based practice for the field of mental health. I will initially examine the traditions of using evidence within the individual mental health disciplines and then describe the development of evidence-based practice in mental health care, mentioning along the way some of the misunderstandings about evidence-based practice and obstacles to its implementation.

The research and practice background

In this section, I will briefly examine the current use of research findings in clinical practice by psychiatrists, psychologists and mental health nurses.

There has always been a strong research background in the fields of psychology, psychiatry and mental health care: from the early descriptive psychopathologists in the nineteenth and early twentieth centuries onwards, there has been an enormous amount of published research in its broadest sense. From an early stage, however, there have been competing schools of thought that start from more or less clearly defined ideological positions and use research to back up their own viewpoints. Throughout its history, psychiatry has been characterised by ideology and controversy about the nature and optimal treatment of mental illness. Perhaps because of this, psychiatry was one of the first medical specialties to undertake randomised controlled trials (RCTs) (National Institute of Mental Health Psychopharmacology Service Center Collaborative Study Group 1964; Medical Research Council 1965).

Archie Cochrane stated that psychiatry was basically inefficient (Cochrane 1989). He argued that there were too many treatments used, too many of which were of uncertain efficacy. But even writing in the 1970s, Cochrane admitted that this had not always been the case, and that progress in the 1950s had shown that psychiatry was in the vanguard of developing empirically based treatment. Clearly, something went wrong.

Psychiatry

There have been few studies of the use of research findings by psychiatrists. However, Smith has reviewed the evidence on information needs of doctors in general (Smith 1996). He concluded that a conservative estimate is that every consultation generates at least one question, and that doctors are most likely to seek the answers to their questions from other doctors. Although there is an enormous amount of clinically relevant information, it is overwhelming because it is disorganised. For *Evidence-Based Mental Health*, (see below) over 5500 potentially relevant journal articles are read every year. To accomplish this him or herself, a clinician would have to read 15 articles each and every day every year (Geddes *et al.* 1999). If the clinician only managed to read two articles every day, after two years, the clinician would have a 10-year backlog. After 20 years, the backlog would take over 100 years to read!

Some of these problems in keeping up to date with research are likely to explain observations of significant variations in clinical practice, even in areas where RCT evidence exists (see Box 4.1).

As has been pointed out, variations in clinical practice can have only two interpretations: either clinicians vary in how they use the results of research in clinical practice or there is no evidence to support their interventions (Kendell 1997).

> ## Box 4.1: Documented variations in clinical practice in psychiatry
>
> ### Electroconvulsive therapy (ECT)
> In a survey of the use of ECT by 17729 psychiatrists in the US, no ECT use was reported in 115 metropolitan statistical areas. Among the remaining 202 metropolitan statistical areas, annual ECT use varied from 0.4 to 81.2 patients per 10000 population (Hermann *et al.* 1995). In a survey of 35 hospitals and five private clinics in the North East Thames and East Anglian regions of the UK National Health Service, considerable variations were found between hospitals. Routine instrument settings varied fourfold between clinics and there were up to twelvefold differences in usage between districts (Pippard 1992).
>
> ### The prescription of stimulants in childhood attention deficit and hyperactivity disorder
> A survey of prescribing found a significant difference in the rates of use of stimulant medication between states and territories in Australia, and a significant increase in use between 1988 and 1993 in Western Australia and New South Wales. In 1993, an estimated 1.6% of males aged 5–16 years were prescribed stimulants in Western Australia compared to about 0.2% in Victoria and Tasmania (Valentine *et al.* 1996).
>
> ### Treatment of schizophrenia
> The Schizophrenia Patient Outcomes Research Team (PORT) study measured the conformance of routine clinical practice in the treatment in schizophrenia with their treatment guidelines. There was limited conformance with the guidelines especially for psychosocial interventions. There were also variations between patient groups, with younger patients more likely to be offered psychotherapy and vocational rehabilitation and ethnic minority patients more likely to be prescribed higher doses of medication and less likely to be prescribed an antidepressant when depressed (Lehman *et al.* 1998).

Clinical psychology

Research into psychologists' behaviour in mental health care has focused on a somewhat different aspect. The majority of studies have examined the use of research by practising clinical psychologists. This is of particular interest because many academic training programmes for clinical psychologists emphasise the importance of the 'scientist–practitioner' – the clinician who adopts a scientific approach to the identification of the patient's problems, choice and use of therapy, and assessment of outcome. Studies of psychologists' use of research evidence suggest that they have tended not to use the research evidence regularly. For example, in a questionnaire survey of 10% of the members and fellows of the psychotherapy division of the American Psychology Association (Division 29), with a 73% response, therapists reported low rates of research utilisation and stated that they gained their most useful information from experience with clients (Morrow Bradley & Elliott 1986). In a questionnaire survey of clinical psychologists, practitioners read an average of two to four journal articles per month, although they highlighted these as one of the most important sources of knowledge (Cohen 1979). In a follow-up study, Cohen *et al.* interviewed 30 clinical psychologists and found that case discussion with clinical colleagues was the most highly valued source of information (Cohen *et al.* 1986). The reasons for this are not clear, although it has been suggested that the scientific purism taught in clinical psychology graduate programmes engenders a scepticism of research which leads many practitioners to dismiss its relevance to clinical practice (Suinn 1993). It is perhaps understandable that in clinical practice 'empirically-supported methods are routinely ignored in favour of intuition and clinical experience' (Wilson 1997).

Mental health nursing

A systematic review of the nursing research literature found that, although there was a large increase in the number of research papers published by mental health nurses between 1982 and 1992, the total amount of research was relatively small compared to that published by psychiatrists and psychologists (Yonge *et al.* 1997). There may also be a number of specific barriers to overcome in order to increase the implementation of research in clinical nursing practice (McKenna 1995), some of which are discussed further in Chapter 6.

The emergence and development of evidence-based practice in mental health

The evolution of evidence-based practice in health care has occurred over a long period – its originators have traced it back to Paris at the end of the eighteenth century (Sackett *et al.* 1996). Since that time there has been a gradual development in the methodology of health services research with the introduction of the modern form of the medical randomised controlled trial in 1948 and the meta-analysis in 1977 (Medical Research Council 1948; Smith & Glass 1977). In mental health, the Quality Assurance Project of the Royal Australian and New Zealand College of Psychiatrists was one of the first attempts to summarise the evidence for interventions and to make recommendations for practice (Quality Assurance Project 1984). In many ways, evidence-based practice can be seen as simply a further development in this process. However, evidence-based practice can also be seen as a more radical development. It is a coherent and comprehensive system made possible by developments in clinical epidemiology and information technology (Sackett *et al.* 1991). For the first time, the resources are in place to allow the clinician to access the best available evidence in real-time clinical practice. Whereas previously, gaining access to evidence was a lengthy and frustrating process, now information is increasingly easily available. More than ever, with the development of the world-wide web and other resources, patients and consumers of health care are highly informed (and sometimes misinformed) about their disorders and treatments. This means that it is increasingly important for clinicians to remain up to date in their field.

Appearance of the term 'evidence-based practice' in professional journals

Within psychiatry, the first use of the term 'evidence-based' practice appears to have been in Bilsker and Gouldner's article (1995). Here, the authors describe the paradigm shift represented by evidence-based practice – in focusing attention away from scientific authority, and reasoning from basic theoretical mechanisms (either pathophysiological or psychological), towards basing practice on empirical evidence. Further articles have since appeared in *Evidence-Based Medicine* and the *British Journal of Psychiatry* in 1996 and 1997 (Geddes 1996; Geddes & Harrison 1997)

In clinical psychology, the term 'empirically validated therapies' (later 'empirically supported therapies') was introduced by the American Psychological Association's Division 12 task force on the promotion and dissemination of psychological procedures, to imply a similar approach – that is, a preference for evidence-based treatments over reasoning from clinical experience or intuition (e.g. Chambless *et al.* 1996). Wilson (1997) drew attention to the similarities between this approach and that of evidence-based medicine.

Emergence of new evidence-based resources in mental health

Systematic reviews

The recognition of the need for systematic reviews of randomised controlled trials, and the development of the scientific methodology of reviews has been one of the most striking developments in health services research over the last decade. The first UK Cochrane Centre was established in Oxford in 1992 as part of the information systems strategy developed to support the NHS Research and Development Programme; Cochrane centres have since been established in many other countries. Within the Cochrane Collaboration, there are several collaborative review groups in areas of practice relevant to mental health clinicians. The longest established group is the Cochrane Schizophrenia Review Group which has so far published almost 30 systematic reviews. Other relevant groups include the Cochrane Depression, Anxiety and Neurosis Group and the Demential and Cognitive Functioning Group.

Current awareness journals

In 1998, a new journal, *Evidence-Based Mental Health*, was introduced with the aim of improving the availability of high-quality evidence to mental health professionals of all disciplines. *Evidence-Based Mental Health* is one of three similar journals, the other two being *Evidence-Based Medicine* and *Evidence-Based Nursing*. Each of these journals has the aim of bringing clinically relevant advances in research to the attention of clinicians. Research can involve treatment (including specific interventions and systems of care), diagnosis, etiology, prognosis/outcome research, quality improvement, continuing education, and economic evaluation. One of the key features of the three journals is that explicit methodological criteria are used to select articles which are only included if they are both methodologically sound and clinically useful (see Box 4.2). The articles are then summarised in value-added abstracts and a commentary by a clinical expert is added.

Box 4.2: Criteria for selection and review of articles for abstracting in *Evidence-Based Mental Health*

Articles are considered for abstracting if they meet the following criteria:

Basic criteria
- Original or review articles
- In English
- About humans
- About topics that are important to the practice of clinicians in the broad field of mental health.

Studies of prevention or treatment must meet these additional criteria:
- Random allocation of participants to comparison groups
- Follow-up (end-point assessment) of at least 80% of those entering the investigation
- Outcome measure of known or probable clinical importance
- Analysis consistent with study design.

Studies of diagnosis must meet these additional criteria:
- Clearly identified comparison groups, at least one of which is free of the disorder of derangement of interest
- Interpretation of diagnostic standard without knowledge of test result
- Interpretation of test without knowledge of diagnostic standard result
- Diagnostic (gold) standard (e.g. diagnosis according to *Diagnostic and Statistical Manual of Mental Disorders*, 4th edn or *International Classification of Diseases*, 10th revision criteria after assessment by clinically qualified interviewer) preferably with documentation of reproducible criteria for subjectively interpreted diagnostic standard (e.g. report of statistically significant measure of agreement among observers)
- Analysis consistent with study design.

Contd

Box 4.2 *Contd*

Studies of prognosis must meet these additional criteria:
- Inception cohort (first onset or assembled at a uniform point in the development of the disease) of individuals, all initially free of the outcome of interest
- Follow-up of at least 80% of patients until the occurrence of a major study end-point or to the end of the study
- Analysis consistent with study design.

Studies of causation must meet these additional criteria:
- Clearly identified comparison group for those at risk of, or having, the outcome of interest (i.e. randomised controlled trial, quasi-randomised controlled trial, non-randomised controlled trial, cohort analytic study with case-by-case matching or statistical adjustment to create comparable groups, case control study)
- Masking of observers of outcomes to exposures (this criterion is assumed to be met if the outcome is objective); observers of exposures masked to outcomes for case control studies; or masking of subjects to exposure for all other study designs
- Analysis consistent with study design.

Studies of quality improvement and continuing education must meet these additional criteria:
- Random allocation of participants or units to comparison groups
- Follow-up of at least 80% of participants
- Outcome measure of known or probable clinical or educational importance
- Analysis consistent with design.

Studies of economics of health care programmes or interventions must meet these additional criteria:
- The economic question addressed must be based on comparison of alternative diagnostic or therapeutic services or quality improvement strategies
- Activities must be compared on the basis of the outcomes produced (effectiveness) and resources consumed (costs)
- Evidence of effectiveness must be from a study (or studies) that meets the journal criteria for diagnosis, treatment, quality improvement, or a review article
- Results should be presented in terms of the incremental or additional costs and outcomes of one intervention over another
- Where there is uncertainty in the estimates or imprecision in the measurement, as sensitivity analysis should be done.

Review articles must meet these additional criteria:
- An identifiable description of the methods indicating the sources and methods for searching articles
- Statement of the clinical topic and the inclusion and exclusion criteria for selecting articles for detailed review
- At least one article included in the review must meet the above noted criteria for treatment, diagnosis, prognosis, causation, quality improvement, or the economics of health care programmes.

Introduction of key skills into professional training

The development of evidence-based practice has resulted in some significant changes to professional training in mental health professions. For example, from summer 1999, the UK Royal College of Psychiatrists will be including a critical review paper into the membership examination, the main postgraduate professional qualification for psychiatrists (Critical Review Paper Working Party 1997). The aims of the critical review paper will be to examine:

(1) The ability to examine critically a published scientific paper, to assess the validity of the scientific information presented and determine its clinical importance and relevance.
(2) The ability to describe logically and clearly the results of such critical appraisal and the processes involved.
(3) The capacity to suggest further experiments that would confirm and/ or expand understanding in the field under investigation.
(4) The ability to place information derived from a piece of research into context in the light of current views and practice.

The knowledge required of candidates will therefore include knowledge of clinical epidemiology, biostatistics and critical appraisal – all of which are central skills of evidence-based medicine. The adoption of the critical review paper is one of the most unequivocal recognitions of the central importance of skills in evidence-based medicine by any of the UK medical royal colleges.

Research training has always been a core feature of the training of UK clinical psychologists. However, research training has focused on producing clinicians who will have the skills to *conduct* clinical research. The development of evidence-based practice has highlighted another important style of research training in which the aim is to provide the skills clinicians need to be able to *use* the results of research in their clinical work. In addition, the recognition of the importance of using empirically supported psychotherapies has major implications for training in clinical psychology (Calhoun *et al.* 1998). One of the advantages of this approach is that some of the sophisticated training materials developed for randomised controlled efficacy studies can be used in training. In the USA, clinical psychology training programmes have begun to emphasise the importance of achieving competence in empirically supported psychotherapies and, by extension, of understanding about research design (Calhoun *et al.* 1998).

The Centre for Evidence-Based Mental Health

The Centre for Evidence-Based Mental Health was founded in Oxford in 1988, with the following aims:

- to promote and support the teaching and practice of evidence-based practice and clinical epidemiology in psychiatry and mental health care throughout the UK and internationally
- to coordinate a national network for clinical effectiveness in mental health (including training, primary research, secondary research, dissemination and audit) in the UK to allow the most effective use of skills and resources
- to initiate a series of large-scale, pragmatic clinical trials in psychiatry.

Initially, the centre has developed a website (URL: http://www.cebmh.com) containing resources for evidence-based practice in mental health. The website also hosts the electronic version of *Evidence-Based Mental Health*.

The development of evidence-based practice in mental health

One aim of evidence-based practice in mental health is to reduce unnecessary variations in clinical practice. Where good evidence for effectiveness already exists this evidence should be reflected in the development and delivery of mental health services. The following section outlines two areas of practice which currently have the potential to be influenced by clinically important evidence.

What is the best model of community care?

In 1991, the UK government introduced a new approach to organising the care of patients with mental disorders, the Care Programme Approach. The Care Programme Approach meant that provider units were required 'to initiate, in collaboration with local social services departments, explicit individually tailored care programmes for all in-patients about to be discharged from mental illness hospitals, and for all new patients accepted by the specialist psychiatric services' (Department of Health 1994). One of the key aims of the Care Programme Approach was to ensure that community care was coordinated and effective, improving patient outcomes and reducing the need for in-patient treatment. The central intervention of CPA was care management, a system in which there is a named key worker who is responsible for:

- assessing the patient's needs – psychiatric, medical and social – as well as risk assessment
- identifying which person or agency is best placed to meet which need
- drawing up a written care plan
- coordinating and reviewing the care plan.

Case management may sound like a very sensible approach to the organisation of community services for severely mentally ill patients. However, the Care Programme Approach was designed and described without any explicit or systematic reference to any evidence for the effectiveness of case management. The approach had apparent validity and the clinical experts advising the government thought it was the best approach. However, when the evidence for the effectiveness of case management compared to standard care was reviewed, it was found to double the rate of admissions to hospital (OR, or odds ratio, 1.84; 99% CI, confidence interval, 1.33–2.57; see Fig. 4.1), with no effect on the clinical or social functioning of the patients, although it did reduce the rate of loss to follow-up (Marshall *et al.* 1996). The results of this review make an interesting contrast with another review of Assertive Community Treatment (ACT), an alternative model of community care that differs from case management in several ways:

- it is more intensive than case management; each team member has fewer patients under their care but is more involved
- the team meet more of the person's needs themselves (rather than involving other agencies)
- responsibility for the patient's care is held collectively by the community mental health team
- it is highly focused on patients with severe psychiatric disorder (especially psychosis) who have a history of multiple admissions or failure to engage and remain in treatment.

A systematic review of ACT found that it decreased admission to hospital by about 40% (Marshall & Lockwood 1998) (OR = 0.59, 99% CI = 0.41–0.85; see Fig. 4.1).

Interpretation of these findings for UK practice requires consideration of all the factors which may limit the generalisability of the findings. Most of the trials were done in countries other than the UK and this may be important – especially as standard care may differ dramatically between countries. It is possible that the size of the effect compared to standard care may be less in the UK – largely because of the provision of the Care Programme Approach. However, the key question is perhaps which model of care is most likely to achieve the desired outcome of a reduction in admission to hospital and a reduction in the duration of stay? On the basis of the best available evidence, it is difficult to avoid the conclusion that ACT is the better form of care delivery. This demonstrates how evidence-based methods could be used to inform policy decisions in a way that has not happened so far. At the time of writing, the UK government has announced a major revision of community mental health services with an apparent intention to make such provisions evidence-based.

(a)

Comparison: CASE MANAGEMENT vs STANDARD CARE
Outcome: Admitted to hospital during study

Study	Expt n/N	Ctrl n/N	Peto OR (95%CI Fixed)	Weight %	Peto OR (95% CI Fixed)
Curtis-New York	48/147	22/145		22.0	2.60 [1.52,4.45]
Ford-London	17/39	14/38		7.7	1.32 [0.53,3.26]
Franklin-Houston	62/213	38/204		31.4	1.77 [1.13,2.78]
Macias-Utah	0/20	6/21		2.2	0.11 [0.02,0.59]
Marshall-Oxford	17/40	10/40		7.5	2.17 [0.86,5.44]
Tyrer-London	58/196	35/197		29.3	1.92 [1.21,3.06]
Total (95% CI)	202/655	125/645		100.0	1.84 [1.43,2.37]

Chi-square 12.88 (df = 5) Z = 4.77

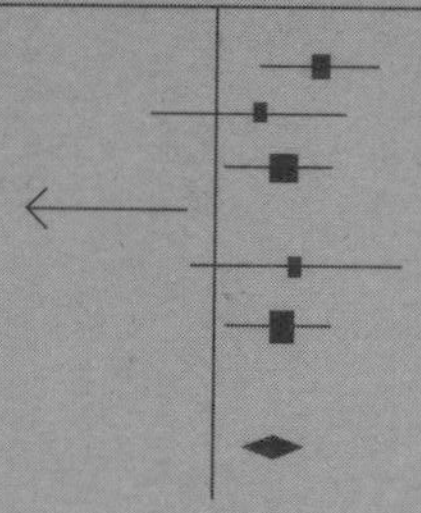

(b)

Comparison: ACT vs STANDARD CARE
Outcome: Admitted to hospital during study

Study	Expt n/N	Ctrl n/N	OR (95%CI Fixed)	Weight %	OR (95% CI Fixed)
Bond-Indiana1	12/50	33/53		18.4	0.19 [0.08,0.45]
Bond-Chicago1	32/45	34/43		7.6	0.65 [0.25,1.73]
Test-Wisconsin	15/75	26/47		19.4	0.20 [0.09,0.45]
Audini-London	9/33	9/33		5.0	1.00 [0.34,2.95]
Lehman-Baltimore	42/77	45/75		15.7	0.80 [0.42,1.52]
Chandler-California	49/252	57/264		34.0	0.88 [0.57,1.34]
Total (95% CI)	159/532	204/515		100.0	0.60 [0.45,0.79]

Chi-square 18.54 (df = 5) Z = 3.68

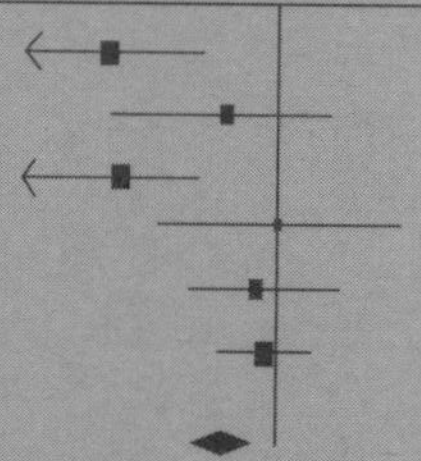

Fig. 4.1   (a) Effectiveness of case management compared to standard care (Marshall *et al.* 1996); and (b) effectiveness of assertive community treatment compared to standard care (Marshall *et al.* 1998).

The growing pains of psychotherapy

The report of the American Psychological Association's Division 12 task force on promotion and dissemination of psychological procedures responded to intense social, economic and political forces to identify which psychological treatments were supported by high-quality evidence. Treatment methods which meet explicit criteria were identified and called collectively 'empirically supported therapies' (Chambless & Hollon 1998). The idea of empirically supported therapies overlaps with the general concept of evidence-based practice in that it proposes that the aim of clinicians is to use the most effective form of treatment for any specific disorder. In addition, the criteria used to classify treatments as empirically supported is a useful step towards developing a critical appraisal tool for using on randomised controlled trials of psychotherapy (Box 4.3). These criteria are similar to other attempts to devise hierarchies of evidence for the effectiveness of treatments (Box 4.4).

Box 4.3: Chambless and Hollon criteria

Comparison with a no treatment control group, alternative treatment group, or placebo: (a) in a randomised controlled trial, controlled single-case experiment, or equivalent time-samples (EST) design and; (b) in which the EST is statistically superior to no treatment, placebo, or alternative treatments or in which EST is equivalent to a treatment already established in efficacy, and power is sufficient to detect moderate differences:

(1) These studies must have been conducted with (a) a treatment manual or its logical equivalent; (b) a population, treated for specified problems, for whom inclusion criteria have been delineated in a reliable, valid manner; (c) reliable and valid outcome assessment measures, at minimum tapping the problems targeted for change; and (d) appropriate data analysis.

(2) For a designation of efficacious, the superiority of the EST must have been shown in at least two independent research settings (sample size of three or more at each site in the case of single-case experiments). If there is conflicting evidence, the preponderance of the well-controlled data must support the EST's efficacy.

(3) For a designation of possibly efficacious, one study (sample size of three or more in the case of single-case experiments) suffices in the absence of conflicting evidence.

(4) For a designation of efficacious and specific, the EST must have been shown to be significantly superior to pill or psychological placebo or to an alternative *bona fide* treatment in at least two independent treatment settings. If there is conflicting evidence, the preponderance of the well-controlled data must support the EST's efficacy and specificity.

Chambless & Hollon 1998

Box 4.4: A hierarchy of evidence used in evidence-based health care

(1)   Strong evidence from at least one systematic review of multiple well-designed randomised controlled trials.

(2)   Strong evidence from at least one properly designed randomised controlled trial of appropriate size.

(3)   Evidence from well-designed trials without randomisation, single group pre-post, cohort, time series or matched case-control studies.

(4)   Evidence from well-designed non-experimental studies from more than one centre or research group.

(5)   Opinions of respected authorities, based on clinical evidence, descriptive studies or reports of expert committee.

Gray 1998

There is also a key difference between empirically supported therapies and evidence-based practice. This concerns methods for the dissemination of research evidence to clinicians. The identification of empirically supported treatments is revised periodically using the criteria to identify additional treatments for which research evidence is positive. Updates to treatment lists are published annually and made available to clinicians through their professional organisation (the American Psychological Association). However, the empirically supported therapies have not yet begun to use information technology resources to increase clinicians' access to clinically important research.

The identification of empirically supported therapies met with outrage from some US clinical psychologist practitioners. Their criticisms have been summarised by Beutler (1998) as follows:

(1)   An unrepresentative and small number of studies constituted the basis of the review.

(2)   The restrictive criteria misrepresented the broad range of research findings.

(3)   Overreliance on studies that used manualised therapies and random assignment led to inaccurate conclusions about the nature of psychotherapy and its effects.

(4)   The findings were likely to be misused both by managed health care and training institutions to limit practice, training or reimbursement to therapies favoured by academicians.

(5)   Any conclusions beyond the general one that generic psychotherapy is effective are premature.

Beutler goes on to state:

> 'Although I am no devotee of randomised controlled trials, manualisation, those criteria originally defined by the Task Force, or even of the assumption that there are diagnosis-specific treatments, I have become convinced that many of the criticisms are overdetermined and nonobjective. The exaggerated reactions tend to cloud, rather than clarify the issues, and leave the impression that the ineffectiveness of one's favourite viewpoint will be found out.'
>
> (Beutler 1998)

A debate between the supporters and critics of empirically supported therapies was published in a special issue of the *Journal of Consulting and Clinical Psychology* (e.g. Kendall 1998). Throughout the issue, there appears to be a growing recognition that, despite their obvious drawbacks, there is no obvious challenge to the RCT as the best way of estimating the efficacy of a treatment, although applying the results in the real world requires a good measure of clinical judgement. Again, this sounds much like the definition of evidence-based medicine: 'conscientious, explicit and judicious use of the current best evidence in making decisions about the care of individual patients' (Sackett *et al.* 1996).

The issue seems to represent a cautious acceptance of the importance of the concept of clinical effectiveness and the need for evidence-based practice. The report of the task force was published in 1998 complete with a forward by Martin Seligman cautioning against 'efficacy imperialism' and including legal disclaimers (Anonymous 1998). The report itself consists of a series of reviews of treatments for a wide range of mental disorders. That they are not methodologically explicit systematic reviews is perhaps not the most important feature of this report; rather, it represents the explicit acceptance of the importance of basing practice on good quality evidence.

A similar process has also occurred in the UK (Parry 1992). A review of the effectiveness of psychotherapy was commissioned by the NHS Executive (Roth & Fonagy 1996; NHS Executive 1996). Relative to the outrage prompted by the introduction of the concept of empirically supported therapies in the USA, the response to the promotion of evidence-based practice in psychotherapy in the UK appears to have been cautious, but positive.

Responses to evidence-based practice

As will be seen from the previous section, evidence-based practice is already having a major impact on mental health services. However, as described, there are also a number of concerns about possible limitations and even dangers of the approach:

(1) *Evidence-based health care is nothing new – good clinicians have always tried to keep up to date with the best available evidence*

Although this may be true, the simple fact is that the voluminous primary research literature meant that is was almost impossible for a clinician to be confident that he or she was completely up to date with the literature. The literature reviewed earlier in the chapter suggests that in many instances, even if they tried, mental health clinicians were unable to keep up to date. Although the aims of evidence-based practice may be the same as those of all good clinicians, evidence-based practice provides a coherent set of strategies to enable the clinician to rapidly identify best knowledge. With the advances in information technology, it is becoming possible to find the required information quickly enough to be clinically useful. The plain fact is that this technology simply was not available until a few years ago.

(2) *There's no evidence that evidence-based health care leads to better patient outcomes*

There is concern that evidence-based practice might not actually lead to better outcomes, or worse still, it might even lead to a lower quality service by encouraging the use of therapies for which there is RCT evidence and discouraging the use of therapies and interventions for which there is no evidence. In order for a drug to be licensed, there needs to be RCT evidence of its effectiveness – this is not the case for non-pharmacological treatments. Because pharmaceutical companies are required to evaluate new drug treatments and because there are profits to be made from new or improved drug treatments, there exists both the means and the motivation to provide evidence of efficacy from RCTs. In contrast, new 'talking' therapies are unregulated, emerge more spontaneously from clinical practice, and are unlikely to generate significant profit for their developers. For these reasons there is no structure within which the means or the motivation exist to provide systematic evaluation of non-pharmacological interventions. Overreliance on treatments for which there is good RCT evidence may therefore lead to overuse of drugs at the expense of non-drug therapies. This is clearly a realistic concern when evaluating older treatments. For new treatments of any kind, there should be a standard level of required evidence – good quality RCTs – before the treatment is widely adopted. This, of course, requires that there is adequate funding for studies of non-drug interventions.

A related issue is that there needs to be clarification of where the responsibility lies for demonstrating clinically meaningful effectiveness of drug treatments. At present, the evidence-based clinician often has to rely on phase III efficacy studies performed by the pharmaceutical industry for the purposes of licensing. These studies are usually based on highly selected samples of patients and are of short duration. It can be difficult to know how the results apply to real-life clinical practice. In the UK, the NHS Research and Development Health Technology Assessment Programme is designed to identify the areas where research is needed and invite applications for funding of research in these areas (Stein & Milne 1999).

(3) There is no evidence in the field of mental health, so there is no point looking

Anecdotally, this is a common belief among the public, who are confused by the enormous number of psychotherapies available and the seeming inability of mental health professionals to prevent the occasional high-profile act of homicide by a mentally ill patient. One reason for the suspicion in which evidence-based practice is held by some practitioners is that there is no evidence to support their practice, and that by drawing attention to this fact evidence-based practice will give purchasers of health care a reason to disinvest in their service. This anxiety is understandably more acute in those disciplines which have a particular allegiance to a single form of therapy. In general, it seems understandable that highly specialist clinicians like psychotherapists are likely to feel particularly at risk.

This tendency to ignore research may be especially marked in psychiatry because of the beliefs and attitudes of the public and even of other clinicians (for example, GPs) regarding mental health and its practitioners (Kerr *et al.* 1995; Priest *et al.* 1996). In fact there is an extraordinary amount of evidence in the field of mental health care. Perhaps because of the continuous interdisciplinary rivalry, practitioners and researchers of various disciplines have not been slow to undertake research on their interventions. It has been found that the proportion of treatment decisions in psychiatry which are based on RCT evidence is similar to that observed in general medicine (Ellis *et al.* 1995; Geddes *et al.* 1996; Summers & Kehoe 1996). However, it was also reported that the quality of the clinical trials was low (Geddes *et al.* 1996).

This profusion of evidence of variable quality leads to difficulties in clinical interpretation. It is clear that bias exists in the research, especially in the form of allegiance bias where researchers who have developed a particular form of therapy are more likely to find that it is effective and better than rival treatments. A particular example is the controversy that surrounds the comparative studies of pharmacological and psychological treatment of depression. Several meta-analyses of drug therapy in depression have been performed to explore the effect of investigator bias on the apparent effect of antidepressants (Greenberg *et al.* 1992; Moncrieff *et al.* 1998). To do this, inevitably, a rather selective and idiosyncratic group of primary studies need to be drawn up which makes the interpretation of these meta-analyses very difficult (Quitkin & Klein 1998). On the other hand, proponents of drug therapy have explained away the apparent equivalence (and possibly superiority) of cognitive therapy as bias in the form of inadequate psychopharmacological control or patient selection (Jacobson & Hollon 1996). It has also apparently been shown, again by meta-analysis of comparative studies, that there is evidence of allegiance bias in the studies showing superiority of cognitive–behaviour therapy over other treatments (Gaffan *et al.* 1995). The result is that for the practising clinician, at present, it is very hard to assess the relative effectiveness of the two treatment modalities.

This example demonstrates one of the problems facing the clinician attempting to use the research evidence. However, in beginning to use the evidence, clinicians can also identify areas of substantial clinical uncertainty where there is insufficient reliable evidence. These areas of clinical uncertainty then become areas of high priority for further research (Geddes 1999). In several countries, there now exist mechanisms for feeding these clinical questions into national health technology assessment programmes, with the objective of ensuring that the allocation of limited research funds are prioritised according to need (Stein & Milne 1999).

(4) Evidence-based practice is only concerned with RCTs which do not answer most clinical questions and which cannot be applied to real-life settings

There are two components to this objection to evidence-based practice. The first of these is the concern that evidence-based practice is only concerned with randomised controlled trials.

Choosing the right research design for a clinical question

The RCT often seems to be considered an overly biomedical form of research design (even though it was first introduced in the field of agriculture), and is resisted because some disciplines may have a research tradition derived more from the social sciences, where the limitations of quantitative research are highlighted and qualitative approaches are preferred. This tension has existed in mental health for decades – and in some ways is analogous to the arguments against positivism in mental health of the 1960s and 1970s.

In fact, evidence-based health care makes no such claims for the universal pre-eminence of the randomised controlled trial for answering all types of clinical questions. Rather, the goal of evidence-based practice is to identify the study design best suited to providing the least biased answer possible to a question. In clinical practice, there are several types of clinical question which commonly arise (see Box 4.5). The research design which is best suited to answering each of these clinical questions may vary (see Box 4.6).

So, while the randomised controlled trial is believed to be the best way of assessing the relative efficacy of a treatment, it is certainly no good for helping a clinician understand what a patient feels about their illness.

Box 4.5: Classification of clinical questions

(1) *Clinical evidence* – how to gather clinical findings properly and interpret them soundly, e.g. when does an idea become delusional? How do we distinguish a true hallucination from a pseudohallucination?

(2) *Diagnosis* – what diagnostic significance do individual clinical phenomena have, e.g. how likely is the diagnosis to be schizophrenia when there is a clear-cut Schneiderian first rank symptom? How useful are screening tests for identifying cases of depressive disorder or alcohol dependence?

(3) *Therapy* – how to select treatments that do more harm than good.

(4) *Prognosis* – how to anticipate the likely course of the patient's illness.

(5) *Education* – how to teach yourself, the patient and the family about the illness, treatment and prognosis.

(6) *Understanding the patient* – how to understand the patient's understanding of the mental health problem.

Sackett *et al.* 1997

Box 4.6: Best research architectures for answering different kinds of clinical question

(1) *Clinical evidence* – intra- and inter-rater reliability study.

(2) *Diagnosis* – cross-sectional study.

(3) *Therapy* – randomised evidence.

(4) *Prognosis* – cohort study of representative patients, inception cohort.

(5) *Education* – randomised evidence.

(6) *Etiology* – randomised, cohort study, case-control study.

Sackett *et al.* 1997

Efficacy and effectiveness

Efficacy and effectiveness are both used as terms for describing how well a treatment achieves its desired outcome: *efficacy* refers to how well a treatment performs in ideal situations – for example in a carefully controlled clinical trial; *effectiveness* describes how well a treatment does in the real world. One of the criticisms of using results of randomised controlled trials in clinical practice is that the findings cannot be applied to the real world, because the participants in trials may be more selected, have less co-morbidity, and have better prognoses and so on. There is obviously some truth in this and a number of strategies have been devised to make the results of randomised controlled trials more applicable in real-life clinical practice. Perhaps the most attractive way is to ensure that trials are *pragmatic*, that is, they reflect the real world by including more representative patients (improving the *external validity* of the trial), while recognising that trial patients are probably never going to be strictly representative of all patients (Sackett & Gent 1979; Simon *et al.* 1995). One of the challenges for researchers will be to ensure that future trials have adequate external validity without compromising internal validity. An alternative way is to extrapolate the findings of efficacy studies using data from representative cohorts of patients (Cook & Sackett 1995).

As well as using the results of randomised controlled trials to estimate the *predicted* effectiveness of treatments, the *observed* effectiveness of treatments can be assessed in representative cohorts of patients. This *outcomes* research is very attractive to the purchasers of health care who want to measure the relative performance of clinicians and clinical services. The relationship between efficacy and effectiveness can be summarised as follows: before using a treatment, we need to know that it is efficacious; we then need to know that it is effective in a particular clinical setting. There is little point trying to estimate the effectiveness of treatments that have not been shown to be efficacious. The advantage of a clinical trial that has both good internal and external validity is that it gives reasonable estimates of both efficacy and effectiveness. Increasingly, there is a recognition that large simple randomised clinical trials that include large numbers of heterogeneous patients and measure clinically meaningful and clear-cut outcomes are likely to provide the most reliable evidence about treatments (Peto *et al.* 1993).

Conclusion

In the past, there appears to have been a considerable gap between research and practice. There now appears to be a growing acceptance that mental health services need to be based on the best available evidence. Evidence-based practice provides an evolving set of strategies which will help clinicians to base their practice on the best available evidence and there are signs that it is being adopted to varying degrees by several professional groups. A major challenge will be to convince sceptical practitioners that the adoption of the evidence-based approach is likely help them to provide the best possible treatment for their patients and to argue effectively for new resources.

Finally, one of the most exciting promises of evidence-based practice is that, by adopting a common approach to the evaluation of treatments and evidence about the effectiveness of treatments, it will be possible for clinicians from all disciplines to transcend some of the interdisciplinary rivalries and to work together to provide the best treatments for their patients.

References

Beutler L.E. (1998) Identifying empirically supported treatments: what if we didn't? *Journal of Consulting and Clinical Psychology*, **66**, 113–20.

Bilsker D. & Goldner E.M. (1995) Evidence-based psychiatry. *Canadian Journal of Psychiatry*, **40**, 97–101.

Calhoun K.S., Moras K., Pilkonis P.A. & Rehm L.P. (1998) Empirically supported treatments: implications for training. *Journal of Consulting and Clinical Psychology*, **66**, 151–62.

Chambless D.L., Sanderson W.C., Shoham V., Bennett Johnson S., Pope K.S. *et al.* (1996) An update on empirically supported therapies. *The Clinical Psychologist*, **49**, 1–8.

Chambless D.L. & Hollon S.D. (1998) Defining empirically supported therapies. *Journal of Consulting and Clinical Psychology*, **66**, 7–18.

Cochrane A.L. (1989) *Effectiveness and Efficiency. Random Reflections on Health Services.* Nuffield Provincial Hospitals Trust, London.

Cohen L.H. (1979) The research readership and information source reliance of clinical psychologists. *Professional Psychology*, **(Dec)**, 780–85.

Cohen L.H., Sargent M.M. & Sechrest L.B. (1986) Use of psychotherapy research by professional psychologists. *American Psychologist*, **(Feb)**, 198–206.

Cook R.J. & Sackett D.L. (1995) The number needed to treat: a clinically useful measure of treatment effect. *British Medical Journal*, **310**, 452–4. Published erratum in *British Medical Journal*, **310**, 1056.

Critical Review Paper Working Party (1997) MRCPsych Part II examination: proposed Critical Review Paper. *Psychiatric Bulletin*, **21**, 381–2.

Department of Health (1994) *The Health of the Nation. Key Area Handbook: Mental Illness* (2nd edition). HMSO, London.

Eccles M., Freemantle N. & Mason J. (1998) North of England evidence-based guidelines development project: methods of developing guidelines for efficient drug use in primary care. *British Medical Journal*, **316**, 1232–5.

Ellis J., Mulligan I., Rowe J. & Sackett D.L. (1995) Inpatient general medicine is evidence based. A-Team, Nuffield Department of Clinical Medicine. *Lancet*, **346**, 407–10.

Gaffan E.A., Tsaousis I. & Kemp Wheeler S.M. (1995) Researcher allegiance and meta-analysis: the case of cognitive therapy for depression. *Journal of Consulting and Clinical Psychology*, **63**, 966–80.

Geddes J. (1996) On the need for evidence-based psychiatry. *Evidence-Based Medicine*, **1**, 199–200.

Geddes J. (1999) Asking structured clinical questions: essential first step of evidence-based practice. *Evidence-Based Mental Health*, **2**, 35–6.

Geddes J.R., Game D., Jenkins N.E., Peterson L.A., Pottinger G.R. & Sackett D.L. (1996) What proportion of primary psychiatric interventions are based on randomised evidence? *Quality in Health Care*, **5**, 215–17.

Geddes J.R. & Harrison P.J. (1997) Evidence-based psychiatry: closing the gap between research and practice. *British Journal of Psychiatry*, **171**, 220–25.

Geddes J.R., Wilczynski N., Reynolds S., Szatmari P. & Streiner D.L. (1999) Evidence-based mental health – the first year. *Evidence-Based Mental Health*, **2**, 3–5.

Gray J.A.M. (1998) *Evidence-Based Healthcare: How to Make Health Policy and Management Decisions*. Churchill Livingstone, New York.

Greenberg R.P., Bornstein R.F., Greenberg M.D. & Fisher S. (1992) A meta-analysis of antidepressant outcome under 'blinder' conditions. *Journal of Consulting and Clinical Psychology*, **60**, 664–9.

Hermann R.C., Dorwart R.A., Hoover C.W. & Brody J. (1995) Variation in ECT use in the United States. *American Journal of Psychiatry*, **152**, 869–75.

Jacobson N.S. & Hollon S.D. (1996) Prospects for future comparisons between drugs and psychotherapy: lessons from the CBT-versus-pharmacotherapy exchange. *Journal of Consulting and Clinical Psychology*, **64**, 104–108.

Kendall P.C. (1998) Empirically supported psychological therapies. *Journal of Consulting and Clinical Psychology*, **66**, 3–6.

Kendell R.E. (1997) The College and 'clinical effectiveness'. *Psychiatric Bulletin*, **21**, 385–6.

Kerr M., Blizard R. & Mann A. (1995) General practitioners and psychiatrists: comparison of attitudes to depression using the depression attitude questionnaire. *British Journal of General Practice*, **45**, 89–92.

Lehman A.F. & Steinwachs D.M. (1998) Patterns of usual care for schizophrenia: initial results from the Schizophrenia Patient Outcomes Research Team (PORT) Client Survey. *Schizophrenia Bulletin*, **24**, 11–20.

Marshall M., Gray A., Lockwood A. & Green R. (1996) Case management for people with severe mental disorders. In C. Adams, J. Anderson & J. de Jesus Mari (eds) *Schizophrenia Module*. Update Software, Oxford.

Marshall M. & Lockwood A. (1998) Assertive community treatment in the care of people with severe mental illness. In *The Cochrane Library*. Update Software, Oxford.

McKenna H.P. (1995) Dissemination and application of mental health nursing research. *British Journal of Nursing*, **4**, 1257–63.

Medical Research Council (1948) Streptomycin treatment of pulmonary tuberculosis. *British Medical Journal*, **(4582)**, 769–73.

Medical Research Council (1965) Clinical trial of the treatment of depressive illness. *British Medical Journal*, **1**, 881–6.

Moncrieff J., Wessely S. & Hardy R. (1998) Meta-analysis of trials comparing antidepressants with active placebos. *British Journal of Psychiatry*, **172**, 227–31.

Morrow Bradley C. & Elliott R. (1986) Utilization of psychotherapy research by practicing psychotherapists. *American Psychologist*, **41**, 188–97.

Nathan P.E. & Gorman J.M. (1998) (eds) *A Guide to Treatments that Work*. Oxford University Press, London.

NHS Executive (1996) *NHS Psychotherapy Services in England*. Department of Health, London.

National Institute of Mental Health Psychopharmacology Service Center Collaborative Study Group (1964) Phenothiazine treatment in acute schizophrenia. *Archives of General Psychiatry*, **10**, 246–61.

Parry G. (1992) Improving psychotherapy services: applications of research, audit and evaluation. *British Journal of Clinical Psychology*, **31**, 3–19.

Peto R., Collins R. & Gray R. (1993) Large-scale randomized evidence: large, simple trials and overviews of trials. *Annals of the New York Academy of Science*, **703**, 314–40.

Pippard J. (1992) Audit of electroconvulsive treatment in two national health service regions [see comments]. *British Journal of Psychiatry*, **160**, 621–37.

Priest R.G., Vize C., Roberts A., Roberts M. & Tylee A. (1996) Lay people's attitudes to treatment of depression: results of opinion poll for Defeat Depression Campaign just before its launch. *British Medical Journal*, **313**, 858–9.

Quality Assurance Project (1984) Treatment outlines for the management of schizophrenia. *Australian and New Zealand Journal of Psychiatry*, **18**, 19–38.

Quitkin F. & Klein D.F. (1998) Antidepressant quandaries. *British Journal of Psychiatry*, **173**, 181.

Roth A.D. & Fonagy P. (1996) *What Works for Whom? A Critical Review of Psychotherapy Research*. Guilford Press, New York.

Sackett D.L. & Gent M. (1979) Controversy in counting and attributing events in clinical trials. *New England Journal of Medicine*, **301**, 1410–12.

Sackett D.L., Haynes R.B., Guyatt G.H. & Tugwell P. (1991) *Clinical Epidemiology: A Basic Science for Clinical Medicine* (2nd edition). Little, Brown and Company, Boston.

Sackett D.L., Richardson S., Rosenberg W. & Haynes R.B. (1997) *Evidence-Based Medicine: How to Practise and Teach EBM*. Churchill-Livingstone, London.

Sackett D.L., Rosenberg W.M., Gray J.A., Haynes R.B. & Richardson W.S. (1996) Evidence-based medicine: what it is and what it isn't [editorial]. *British Medical Journal*, **312**, 71–2.

Sackett D.L. & Wennberg J.E. (1997) Choosing the best research design for each question [editorial]. *British Medical Journal*, **315**, 1636–7.

Simon G., Wagner E. & Vonkorff M. (1995) Cost-effectiveness comparisons using 'real-world' randomized trials: the case of new antidepressant drugs. *Journal of Clinical Epidemiology*, **48**, 363–73.

Smith M.L. & Glass G.V. (1977) Meta-analysis of psychotherapy outcome studies. *American Psychologist*, **32**, 752–60.

Smith R. (1996) What clinical information do doctors need? *British Medical Journal*, **313**, 1062–8.

Stein K. & Milne R. (1999) Mental health technology assessment: practice-based research to support evidence-based practice. *Evidence-Based Mental Health*, **2**, 37–9.

Suinn R.M. (1993) Practice – its not what we preached. *The Behaviour Therapist*, **(Feb)**, 47–9.

Summers A. & Kehoe R.F. (1996) Is psychiatric treatment evidence-based? *Lancet*, **347**, 409–10.

Valentine J., Zubrick S. & Sly P. (1996) National trends in the use of stimulant medication for attention deficit hyperactivity disorder. *Journal of Paediatric Child Health*, **32**, 223–7.

Wilson G.T. (1997) Treatment manuals in clinical practice [comment]. *Behaviour Research and Therapy*, **35**, 205–210.

Yonge O., Austin W., Zgou Qiuping P., Wacko M., Wilson S. & Zaleski J. (1997) A systematic review of the psychiatric/mental health nursing research literature 1982–1992. *Journal of Psychiatric and Mental Health Nursing*, **4**, 171–7.

Chapter 5

Evidence-Based Public Health

J. A. Muir Gray

Introduction

Das Untergang des Abendlandes

The translation of the title of Oswald Spengler's (1991) huge work, *The Decline of the West*, is, as is often the case, less impressive than its original German title (*Das Untergang des Abendlandes*). Spengler's panoramic review of western history portrays a gradual decline in the power and influence of the west and, being written before the rise of Japan and the tiger economies of Asia, his book was much criticised because it seemed at one time that the west, including the USA, had never been more powerful or influential. Powerful though the recent effects of the Asian financial crisis have been, however, the west received a much shorter, sharper shock which brought home only too well its vulnerability and impotence when the Organisation of Global Petroleum Exporting Countries (OPEC) led by Sheikh Yamani caused shock waves by hiking the price of oil dramatically in 1974.

For those managing health care resources the impact was immediate and dramatic because, in addition to the alarming television pictures of cars queuing at petrol pumps, those who were managing health services had to set up systems to do such unimaginable tasks as producing petrol coupons and deciding which staff were, or were not, eligible for these perquisites; district nurses were, quite appropriately, at the top of the list for coupons. The shock waves of the OPEC action also had a longer-term effect, for it strengthened the resolve of Mrs Thatcher's Conservative government to tackle what they saw as decades of complacency and introversion and recreate a vibrant economy with a lean and efficient government. This move in the UK was complemented by changes elsewhere, notably in the USA which, although relatively immune from the OPEC oil crisis, understood globalisation, and also rejected post-war middle-ground politics in favour, not of the socialist left, but of the free-market right, electing Ronald Reagan as president.

Not only did they see the market as a means of solving both economic and social problems, but the policies of Thatcher and Reagan also sought to reduce the size of government. The ideology behind this viewed government as too intrusive into the life of the individual. There were also hard economic reasons, notably that the main factor determining the level of taxation was the size of public expenditure, so reducing taxation to give more people more money to spend necessarily meant a reduction in government income and therefore government expenditure. This led, in the UK although not in the USA, to the imposition of severe constraints on health expenditure, thereby creating one of the first, necessary preconditions for evidence-based decision-making to flourish.

The policy background

To those who worked in the health service, the decades following the OPEC oil crisis were hard years, just how hard is perhaps only remembered by those who had experienced the balmy days of growth in the 1950s and 1960s. For those who have worked in the NHS only since the OPEC oil crisis, times have always been hard; but for those who wished to see a more rational approach adopted in decision-making, the rigour imposed by economic stringency created a climate in which epidemiology moved from an academic environment to health care management and clinical decision-making. In the UK, the second necessary precondition for evidence-based health care also obtained, namely a commitment to cover the whole population.

Professor Alan Enthoven, a Stanford academic, was one of the original 'whizz kids' brought in by Robert Macnamara to revolutionise the management of the Pentagon when he was Secretary for Defense in the Kennedy administration. The heady excitement, optimism and hubris of those years, and its nemesis, is beautifully captured by David Halberstam's (1972) book *The Best and the Brightest*, in which Macnamara emerges as a central figure, confident in the power of his managerial techniques to analyse and systematise the American response to the nuclear arms race. After his time in the Pentagon Alan Enthoven returned to the private sector and academia and became one of the most influential thinkers and advocates of free market reform of western economies. He believed that competition between providers of health care would drive down cost and improve quality, as had happened with many other human activities, notably the production of consumer goods such as the automobile. The suggestion caught the attention of Mrs Thatcher who had grown eager for a radical solution to what seemed to be never-ending resource problems in the NHS. Enthoven's influence was not the only factor, but it was an important element in creating the market reforms which included the divorce of health authorities, who were the 'purchasers', from primary care teams, community care teams and hospitals, who were the 'providers'. The competition between providers failed to materialise with the vigour that the advocates of the internal market had hoped for, but there were two very important consequences which changed the focus and function of health authorities.

The first consequence was that health authorities were freed from the problems of providing health care – namely, they did not have to worry in detail about what went on in hospital wards and primary care teams in the way that they had done before the split. Before the division of purchaser and provider, health authorities had been responsible for, and too often preoccupied by, issues such as industrial relations problems which occupied large amounts of their time and energy.

The second benefit, following on from the first, was that health authorities were required to focus on the needs of populations and to make the best use of finite resources for their populations. This was quite different from the fuzzier arrangements which had formerly applied. Previously money was allocated down the provider line to health authorities which were responsible for both teaching based on often arcane and esoteric funding formulae, and also specialist centres providing tertiary services for an ill-defined population.

Pressure-cooker decision-making and its consequences

As the gap between need and demand, on the one hand, and resources on the other widened because of population ageing, new technology and rising expectations, of both patients and professionals, the pressure on decision-makers, those people responsible for allocating resources to different populations or different groups within the population, became increasingly:

- open
- explicit
- evidence-based.

Consumer pressure leads to a demand for openness in decision-making and this is initially alarming, but decision-makers soon learn that they have little to fear from openness, in part because the press is often more interested in stories about cover-ups than stories about hard choices; and in part because the public have to face up to these hard choices themselves, for they bear some responsibility for the amount of resources allocated to health care and should be involved in decision-making.

Because the competition for the resources available becomes ever tougher, those who bid for new resources and those who fight to defend their service from cuts, both wish and are expected to argue their case explicitly, whereas when resources are more plentiful decisions can be more opaque. As decision-making becomes more explicit, the premises on which decisions are based are set out more clearly and can be scrutinised more easily, and any scrutiny of decision-making may reveal that the propositions can be divided into two types:

- value statements; and
- facts or propositions supported by evidence.

The latter category can be further subdivided into: propositions supported by the evidence of personal experience, sometimes called opinion, and propositions supported by evidence derived from research.

The emergence of evidence-based health care

A number of different disciplines can, of course, contribute evidence to evidence-based decision-making but a number of us with an epidemiological background decided to develop epidemiology for managers as a training programme, supported by the Oxford Regional Health Authority. We defined a number of core competences for managers allocating resources for health care and these are set out in Box 5.1.

A number of training programmes were developed in the early 1980s to help managers acquire these competences and apply them in everyday life. Some of these topics and training programmes focused solely on populations, but we soon found that those who manage health care resources for populations or groups of patients could accept the need for an epidemiological approach, but were still puzzled by clinical practice.

Studies of variations in the level of care provided to similar populations carried out in the US by Jack Wennberg led to a number of similar studies within the UK, and to international comparison (Fullard *et al.* 1984). These studies revealed variations in the rate of intervention much greater than could be explained by variations in need in the different populations, leading to the conclusion that clinical practice was not perhaps as cut-and-dried as the image of modern scientific medicine had suggested.

This was of particular concern to those managers involved in epidemiology training because they could see that, however logical they were when dealing with populations, individual clinicians varied widely in their clinical practice, in adopting new technologies or discarding old and discredited technologies, and that the behaviour of clinicians was of central interest to those who manage resources. As a finance director trenchantly expressed it, 'its the docs who spend the money'. One book, more than any other, helped expose and clarify the science of clinical decision-making, and that book was *Clinical Epidemiology*, appropriately sub-titled *A Basic Science for Clinical Practice*, which expressed and captured the approach

Box 5.1: Core competences for managers allocating resources for health care

Improving quality by increasing appropriateness:

- List the possible reasons for variation in rates of care
- Discuss the relationship between referral rate and quality of care
- Discuss the factors that influence the decision of a GP to refer an individual patient and the referral rate of a GP and a practice
- Define the concept of appropriateness both with respect to individual patients and with respect to groups of patients.

Using the scientific literature to best effect

- Identify randomised controlled trials and systematic reviews in the scientific literature
- Appraise articles on randomised controlled trials and systematic reviews
- Understand the meaning of P values and confidence intervals.

Comparing options

- Define and contrast cost-effectiveness analysis, cost-benefit analysis, and cost-utility analysis
- Define QALYS and describe how they are constructed
- List the strengths and weaknesses of QALYS
- Discuss the ethical issues involved in resource allocation
- Describe a framework that could be used by clinicians to measure the appropriateness of an intervention or service
- Distinguish between effectiveness and appropriateness and define the relationship between these two aspects of quality
- Describe the relationship between variations in rates of intervention and appropriateness and suggest how clinical teams can identify inappropriate use of resources
- Discuss the part played by changing case mix to increase the appropriateness of a service as a whole and thus increase the effectiveness of a service
- Describe interventions that have been demonstrated as being effective in modifying inappropriate referral patterns.

developed in McMaster University (Sackett *et al.* 1985, 1991). McMaster University was an old university in Hamilton, Ontario, with a new medical school which, with very enlightened leadership, decided to adopt a completely new approach to medical education. These old and new approaches are set out in Box 5.2.

McMaster University pioneered new methods of medical education, notably problem-based learning, and recognised early on that those who did or would do research had different educational needs from those who would be primarily users of research findings, with the latter group being more numerous than the former (Fig. 5.1).

Of central importance was the recognition of the fact that scientific

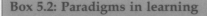

Box 5.2: Paradigms in learning

Old	*New*
● knowing what you *should* know	● knowing what you *don't* know
● much learning 'complete' at the end of formal training	● able to question received wisdom
● apprenticeship, learning from accepted wisdom	● able to generate and refine a question, and to find, appraise, and store, and act on evidence to solve it
● finite amount of knowledge to be absorbed	● life-long learner
● intuition – very powerful	● complementing experience with knowledge from research
● dominated by knowledge from experience	● problem-based learning
● knowledge-based learning	● doctors on tap
● doctors on top	

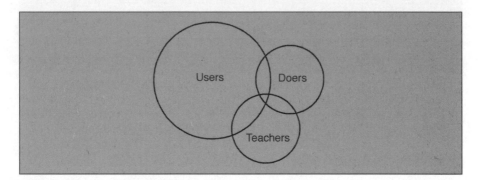

Fig. 5.1   The research constituencies.

journals were written by researchers for researchers, and that the articles published in these journals were of little use to the users, rather than the doers, of research. The users of research findings therefore had to be taught the skills of critical appraisal, and their teachers had to be helped to develop a new approach to teaching.

Developing a new approach for linking science to practice

The appreciation that it was clinicians who spent resources, and that changes in clinical practice were of major importance to those who made macro decisions, was provided with an evidence base by David Eddy (1993). Eddy, one of the leading thinkers in this field, estimated that health care managers and policy-makers in the US, when faced with rising costs, could certainly ascribe some of these costs to forces outside their control, notably population ageing and the general rate of inflation; but that a significant proportion of the remainder, about a third of the total increase in costs, were due to changes in volume and intensity of clinical practice (Fig. 5.2). The type of changes taking place in clinical practice, often imperceptible to managers and sometimes imperceptible to clinicians themselves, are set out in Box 5.3.

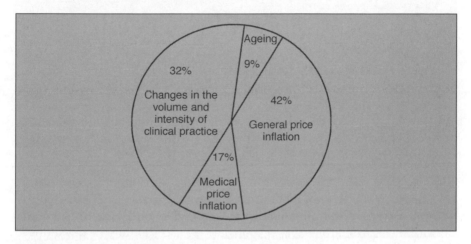

Fig. 5.2 Sources of health expenditure escalation.

The development of evidence-based health care

The House of Lords has been much criticised, but the contribution that a more reflective, less partisan, chamber can make to debate on the development of policy is easy to overlook, and the origins of the NHS Research and Development Programme lie in a report from the House of Lords Select Committee (House of Lords Select Committee on Science and Technology 1987–88). This report pointed out that the research agenda driven by research workers produced information, but did not necessarily produce the answers to the questions posed by patients, clinicians, managers and policy-makers. Furthermore, they pointed out that even if research produced answers that were of relevance to the improvement of the public health, or the management of the health service, or the effectiveness and efficiency of the delivery of health care, there was no system for ensuring that those results were translated into practice.

Based on their recommendations, the Department of Health decided to set

Box 5.3: How innovations in clinical practice increase costs

- Treating conditions that were previously untreatable

- Treating people who would previously have been untreated because of changing professional perceptions of need and appropriateness and changing public expectations. These may result from:
    increasing safety of intervention
    more acceptable, less invasive, more pleasant interventions
    changing attitudes to chronological age as a reason for refusing treatment
    changing expectations about health and disease.

- Providing more expensive types of treatment:
    more expensive drugs
    more expensive imaging
    more expensive tests
    more expensive staff.

- More intensive clinical practice:
    longer duration of stay
    more tests per patient
    more professional interventions per patient
    more treatments per patient.

Eddy 1993

up a research and development programme analogous to, but not identical with, research and development in industry. Obviously the research and development programme was responsible for ascertaining the questions to which decision-makers wanted answers, and ensuring that the answers that were required were produced; but two other important functions were identified for the research and development programme, namely:

- ensuring that there is easy access to knowledge; and
- promoting an evaluative culture.

Improving the availability of knowledge

The McMaster University formula (see Fig. 5.3) indicates that performance is a function of three variables, being directly related to motivation and competence, and inversely related to the barriers that people have to overcome.

$$P = \frac{M \times C}{B}$$

Fig. 5.3 Practitioner performance formula.

Increasing motivation

No attempt was made to motivate people to practise evidence-based decision-making. Indeed, it was known that the adoption of the term evidence-based medicine, developed in the US and Canada in the early 1990s, would irritate a number of people, so that choice of this term for the Centre for Evidence-Based Medicine, and the journal of secondary publication produced by the BMJ Publishing Group, was a calculated risk designed not to motivate people but to raise the profile of a style of decision-making.

The work to create an evaluative culture, described in the following section, did lead to increased motivation but no conscious attempt was made to increase motivation of individuals by exhortation. It was recognised, however, that leadership by example could play a part, and for this reason the recruitment of Professor David Sackett from McMaster University to head the Centre for Evidence-Based Medicine in 1994 was a particularly significant step.

Developing the competence for evidence-based decision-making

The Critical Appraisal Skills Programme (CASP) was developed by Oxford Regional Health Authority to promote the skills needed for critical appraisal. Simple techniques for appraising different scientific methods, and the application of these methods to different problems, were developed and taught in workshops lasting no more than one or two afternoons. An example of a critical appraisal checklist is shown in Box 5.4.

The original intention was to develop cascade training throughout the whole country and it was hoped that departments of public health,

---

Box 5.4: Checklist for appraising review articles

A. Are the results of the review valid?

Screening questions
(1) Did the review address a clearly focused issue?
HINT: An issue can be 'focused' in terms of:
- the population studied
- the intervention given
- the outcomes considered

(2) Did the authors look for the appropriate sort of papers?
HINT: The best sorts of studies would:
- address the review's question
- have an appropriate design study
Is it worth continuing?

Contd

Box 5.4 *Contd*

Detailed questions

(3)   Do you think the important, relevant studies were included?
HINT: Look for:
- which bibliographic databases were used
- follow-up from reference lists
- personal contact with experts
- search for unpublished as well as published studies
- search for non-English language studies

(4)   Did the review's authors do enough to assess the quality of the included studies?
HINT: The authors need to consider the rigour of the studies they have identified. Lack of rigour may affect the studies' results.

(5)   If the results of the review have been combined, was it reasonable to do so?
HINT: Consider whether:
- the results were similar from study to study
- the results of all the included studies are clearly displayed
- the results of the different studies are similar
- the reasons for any variations in results are discussed

B.   What are the results?

(6)   What is the overall result of the review?
HINT: Consider:
- if you are clear about the review's 'bottom line' results
- what these are (numerically if appropriate)
- how were the results expressed (NNT, odds ratio, etc.)

(7)   How precise are the results?
HINT: Look for confidence limits

C.   Will the results help locally?

(8)   Can the results be applied to the local population?
HINT: Consider whether:
- the patients covered by the review could be sufficiently different to your population to cause concern
- your local setting is likely to differ much from that of the review

(9)   Were all important outcomes considered?

(10) Are the benefits worth the harms and costs?
Even if this is not addressed by the review, what do you think?

Source: Gray 1997

including both academic and service departments, would take up the training materials developed by CASP and use them to take the lead in promoting evidence-based decision-making in and for their populations. But there was little evidence that public health departments across the country as a whole saw this as an important function, or as a potential for future development. Accordingly, a move was made to develop open learning materials and place less reliance on the cascade strategy.

It was recognised also that CASP was a form of remedial education and that it was necessary to change curricula for those in basic training so that the need for CASP would, in time, diminish as cohorts of professionals who had received training in finding, appraising and storing knowledge emerged from the training courses.

Knocking down the barriers

The main emphasis given in all of the work to promote evidence-based decision-making was to reduce the barriers. The experience of those running workshops was that the initial reaction by the majority of people who heard about evidence-based medicine was enthusiastic. The definition of evidence-based medicine publicised in a *British Medical Journal* editorial (reproduced in Box 5.5) led to many people appreciating that evidence-based medicine was not 'cookbook' medicine, that it had to incorporate the values and needs of the individual patient, and they would therefore wish to adopt it.

Box 5.5: Definition of evidence-based medicine

Evidence-based medicine in the conscientious, explicit, and judicious use of current best evidence in making decisions about the care of individual patients. The practice of evidence-based medicine means integrating individual clinical expertise with the best available external clinical evidence from systematic research. By individual clinical expertise we mean the proficiency and judgement that individual clinicians acquire through clinical experience and clinical practice (Sackett *et al.* 1996)

What became apparent was that thousands of health care professionals had no easy access to a library, notably those in primary care, mental health and learning disability services, and even those who had access found difficulty in finding the knowledge they needed. A number of steps were taken to make it much easier to find best current knowledge.

The research and development programme promoted the production of systematic reviews, as for the busy clinician or policy-maker finding five, ten or twenty randomised controlled trials (RCTs) often meant they were unable to use this trial data in decision-making because the volume of information was just too great. By producing systematic reviews, particularly those produced by the Cochrane Collaboration, information was distilled into useful knowledge. The key characteristics of a systematic review are described in Box 5.6.

> **Box 5.6: Key characteristics of a systematic review**
>
> **A systematic review:**
>
> - is based on an exhaustive search for all the relevant literature
> - uses explicit and validated criteria for excluding evidence that is of inadequate quality
> - cites the evidence that has been excluded
> - uses valid and explicit methods for combining data, a process called meta-analysis.
>
> These techniques increase the power and decrease the bias of research findings.
>
> **What distinguishes a Cochrane review?**
> Cochrane reviews are produced by the Cochrane Collaboration and are a subset of systematic reviews of the effects of health care which:
>
> - are based on randomised controlled trials
> - always involve consumers in their production
> - are produced to the guidelines in the Cochrane Collaboration Handbook
> - are published in the Cochrane Library.

The practical problems faced by decision-makers in gaining access to best current knowledge, even if it was available, were tackled in a project managed by the Health Care Libraries Unit in Oxford, a unit jointly funded by Oxford University and the regional health authority, known as the Library of the 21st Century Project. The main focus of this was to develop a strategy which would allow clinicians to have access to best current knowledge within 15 seconds. The Oxford Facilitator Scheme in the 1980s had found that for busy clinicians anything that took longer than 30 seconds was unlikely to be done regularly. Based on this evidence it was therefore necessary to produce knowledge that could be read in 15 seconds, after being found in 15 seconds. The Library of the 21st Century Project included the development of the skills of librarians, and the project focused particularly on the needs of those who had most difficulty with gaining access to best current knowledge, namely people working in learning disability, mental health and primary care services. This strategy contributed to the development of ideas that underpin the concept of a national electronic library for health which was included in the recently published *Information for Health* strategy (Department of Health 1998).

Creating an evaluative culture

In the early days of the promotion of evidence-based decision-making, a three-step model which provided the CASP logo was used as the basis for all activities to promote an evidence-based culture. The three steps were:

(1) Find
(2) Appraise
(3) Act.

However, Scott Richardson, who came to Oxford on sabbatical from the University of Rochester to the Centre for Evidence-Based Medicine, and became one of the joint authors of the *Evidence-Based Medicine Handbook* (Sackett *et al.* 1997), added a very significant fourth step by emphasising that before people could find the answer they had to ask the *right* question.

Some skill is needed in asking questions, but what is primarily needed is a change in behaviour, in which decision-makers asked much more frequently the question, 'what is the evidence?'. One reason why this question was seldom asked was because of the difficulty in finding evidence, and therefore the measures described in the previous section would facilitate a change in behaviour. It was, however, decided that a number of steps should be taken to promote an evidence-based decision-making culture. Examples of these initiatives are described below.

GRiPP – getting research into purchasing and practice

Projects were identified in which there was a gap between what was known and what was done, and a wide variety of different measures were adopted to drive the evidence into practice, either to:

- increase the uptake of a cost-effective intervention, e.g. steroids in pre-term labour or aspirin after myocardial infarction; or
- stop an intervention for which there was no good evidence of effectiveness, e.g. D&C operations for younger women with menstrual problems.

Bandolier

Epidemiology perhaps competes with economics for the title of the gloomy science and Oxford Regional Health Authority Research and Development Programme decided to publish *Bandolier*. The name was chosen because of the experience of one of the editors when, as a purchaser, he had felt like the Emperor Maximilian in the famous painting by Manet – standing alone and blindfolded against the hail of bullets from the firing squad. The clinicians seem to have all the bullets and the original objective of *Bandolier* was to write bullets for purchasers, in particular GP fundholders. (Showing how false memory can be unless backed by evidence, it is important to note that, contrary to the conviction of the editor, the Emperor was not blindfolded and the firing squad did not have bandoliers.)

The impact of *Bandolier* has been considerable and many GPs use it as a source of knowledge, even though it was primarily designed to change culture.

Workshops on evidence-based decision-making

A range of different workshops were organised covering either different types of service, for example evidence-based learning disability services, or different professions, for example evidence-based occupational therapy and physiotherapy.

Evidence-based patient and public choice

Perhaps the most radical move to promote evidence-based decision-making was to focus on patients and the public. The CASP programme had already focused on the public, at least representatives of the public such as community health council secretaries, members of maternity liaison committees, and non-executives in health authorities and trusts, and have found that it was possible to create not only the skills of critical appraisal but also the confidence for non-clinicians to ask clinicians, 'what and how good is the evidence?'

Because the consumers were themselves not clear about the way in which clinicians worked, it was felt that the evidence-based medicine programme should focus on evidence-based patient and public choice. Dr Tony Hope was asked to prepare a report on the concept of evidence-based patient choice (Hope 1996).

Evidence-based health care – a UK invention

Evidence-based medicine was developed in the USA and Canada, where clinical epidemiology is traditionally strong. Evidence-based health care, the use of best current knowledge as evidence in decision-making about groups and populations, was, however, a term developed in the UK. In evidence-based health care, decisions about groups and populations are based on best current knowledge. It is important to emphasise the difference between evidence-based clinical practice, the generic term which covers evidence-based decision-making in all clinical specialties, and evidence-based health care.

In the former, based on the definition of evidence-based medicine given in Box 5.5, the needs and values of the individual patient have to be taken into account, together with the evidence. The cost of the intervention was not, however, promoted as a major factor for clinicians to consider. In evidence-based health care, on the other hand, cost or, to be precise, opportunity cost, was regarded as being of central importance and decisions were envisaged as being based on evidence that took into account the needs and values of the population and the resource implications of the decision (Fig. 5.4).

For example, there is evidence that the use of TPA (tissue plasminogen activator) has a small benefit, which is greater than that obtained from streptokinase in the treatment of myocardial infarction. The cost, however, of using TPA is very great. In the UK, and in many other countries now, it is seen that decisions about which interventions should be made available should be made at the level of society, leaving clinicians to make the best use of the resources made available to them. For example, those making a decision for a population could decide there were more valuable ways of spending the additional resources required to add TPA to streptokinase in the range of treatments available for people with myocardial infarction, leaving individual clinicians to make the best use of streptokinase once that decision had been made.

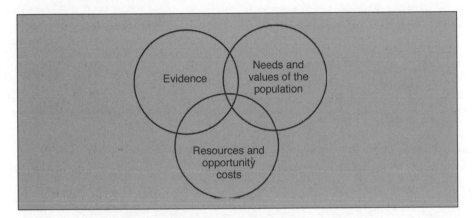

Fig. 5.4   Factors incorporated in evidence-based health care decisions.

Implications for public health

Public health has been at the centre of most of the initiatives described above, and many public health professionals in the UK have made a major contribution to the development of evidence-based clinical practice and evidence-based health care. Public health in the UK, however, is not typical of public health elsewhere in the world because of its close involvement with health care delivery.

The precise contribution that high-quality health care makes to health improvement is still a subject of debate. There is, however, no doubt that good quality health care does make a contribution to the health of populations and it is therefore entirely appropriate for public health professionals to be involved in activities that improve the quality, effectiveness and acceptability of health care. There are, however, critics who say that public health in the UK has spent too much time on this aspect of public health, particularly since the introduction of health care purchasing, and that the opportunity costs of this involvement, as measured by the amount of time that health care professionals could have spent in dealing with other factors which affect the public health, for example poverty and inequality, has been too high. Part of the work that has been done in the last five years has, however, been to promote evidence-based public health, for example through the journal of secondary publication called *Journal of Evidence-Based Health Policy and Management* which publishes structured abstracts of articles of adequate quality in the field of health policy and health care management. An example of a summary in the journal on evidence-based public health is shown in Box 5.7.

Box 5.7: Example of a structured abstract

Evidence-based public health

The tobacco industry is seeking to prevent local communities from taking legal action by pre-emptive legislation at state level.
Siegel M., Carol J., Jordan J., Hobart R., Schoenmarklin S., DeMelle F. & Fisher P. (1997) Pre-emption in tobacco control: review of an emerging public health problem. *Journal of the American Medical Association*, **278**, 858–63.

Background
Legislation is an important and effective public health intervention in smoking control. The tobacco industry is seeking to counter this, particularly by preventing local legislation which is known to be particularly effective.

Objective
To review tobacco control legislation and analyse the relationship between state legislation and actual or potential legislation by local communities.

Setting
USA

Method
A computerised database of community tobacco control ordinances (local legislation), state tobacco control laws, and pre-emption bills introduced during the 1996 state legislative session, were reviewed. The content of the pre-emption bills and the state laws were analysed by multiple observers. The data were then synthesised for the report.

Literature review
Explicit search strategy of local tobacco control ordinances, state laws and the medical literature; 64 references.

Contd

Box 5.7 *Contd*

Results
By the end of 1995, 1006 communities had enacted a local tobacco control ordinance. In 29 states the tobacco industry has now put forward legislation to pre-empt local authority tobacco control through the power to issue a local ordinance. During 1996 alone, 26 bills containing pre-emption clauses were introduced and two were enacted. Emerging trends in the strategy to prevent local tobacco control ordinances were identified, notably:

(1)   Amending legitimate tobacco control bills to pre-empt local tobacco regulations; in this technique the tobacco industry uses a bill prepared by public health advocates; in this approach a bill to prevent, for example, access by young people to cigarette sales, is amended by supporters of the tobacco industry to include pre-emption as well as the beneficial objective of the bill.

(2)   The straight promotion of 'super pre-emption bills' to preclude all local action by community governments on tobacco issues; during the 1996 session, eight of the 26 pre-emption bills that were introduced contained a super pre-emption clause that would have eliminated all local government powers to regulate any aspect of tobacco policy; use of the retail industry to advocate alternative approaches to tobacco control, combined with pre-emptive legislation.

Authors' conclusions
The authors conclude that the tobacco industry is developing a very effective pre-emption strategy and that public health advocates are sometimes insufficiently sophisticated to detect and counter this strategy. They conclude that: 'local control should be viewed as a public health tool that must be protected and all attempts to enact pre-emptive legislation should be fought vigorously by the public health and medical communities'.

Competence and barriers within public health

The basic science on which evidence-based decision-making is based is epidemiology, and public health is ideally positioned to lead work in evidence-based decision-making because it is one of the few disciplines in which epidemiology is one of the basic sciences. However, the competence of public health professionals to teach evidence-based decision-making cannot be assumed and the barriers they have to overcome are considerable.

It is reported that American lawyers have been sued for failing to search the relevant databases sufficiently thoroughly to establish whether or not there was legal precedent for a particular situation. The same could occur in public health in the UK. The vignette below was used to stimulate debate at a workshop on the skills required for evidence-based public health, held in Oxford in December 1995.

Barrister: 'Dr X, perhaps you could tell us a little bit about how you searched for the evidence to support your assertion.'

Dr X: 'Well, I started with MEDLINE and did a full MEDLINE search, and also an Embase search.'

Barrister: (The barrister strikes back) 'But Embase and MEDLINE cover only 7000 of the 20 000 journals in the world; did you look at Psychlit? What steps did you take to look at languages other than English?'

Dr X: 'I plead the Fifth Amendment.'

Barrister: 'Now let us come to appraisal, Dr X. Tell me a little bit about the techniques you used to appraise the cohort studies; in particular I wonder if you could tell me what you think the Mantel-Haenzel approach has to offer in this case?'

The skills required in the management of evidence are the skills of searching, appraising and storing evidence, and the skills required and, where possible, the standards of practice that should be expected of the public health professional, were discussed in the workshop.

SAS skills

For each of the three main skills of searching, appraising and storing a number of components were identified and for some of these it was possible to set measurable levels of performance. These are set out in Boxes 5.8, 5.9 and 5.10.

The public health professional who does not have these skills could plead that their training had been deficient and steps obviously have to be taken to improve training; for example, only a small proportion of public health professionals can use reference management software. However, even if everyone had had the best possible training, resources are required to practise evidence-based decision-making which are not universally

---

Box 5.8: Searching

The decision-maker should be able to:

- describe sources of information other than their local library which they have used when their librarian was not available
- describe at least two databases of relevance to their field of work
- define what is meant by terms commonly used in searching, for example:
  - explode
  - MeSH
  - Boolean operators
- conduct a search using more than one search item, preferably against a gold standard search by a trained searcher.

Box 5.9: Appraisal skills

Every decision-maker should:

- have a set of criteria against which they can appraise the type of research papers they commonly use, for example:
  - systematic reviews
  - randomised trials
  - case control studies
  - cohort studies
  - surveys
- be able to present an appraisal of a research paper which clarified the strengths and weaknesses of the paper
- write a review of a number of papers that they have appraised.

Box 5.10: Storing skills

All professional decision-makers should have a system for storing the knowledge and evidence that is essential to their practice in a way which can be retrieved whatever the reason for the search. They should:

- have, or have access to, a computer-based reference management system
- be able to input individual records to that system
- download the results of a search to their system
- perform searches on their system using more than one search item.

available. Thus the ability to acquire, develop, use and improve the skills of searching, appraising and storing requires databases, the ability to access those databases, and a new form of organisation for public health. These three factors are all prerequisites for evidence-based public health (Fig. 5.5).

Every public health professional has access to the databases set out in Box 5.11.

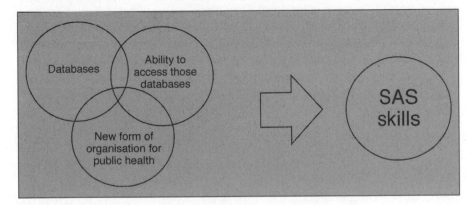

Fig. 5.5 Prerequisites for evidence-based public health.

Box 5.11: Databases

- The Cochrane Database of Systematic Reviews
- The database of reviews of effectiveness produced by the Centre for Reviews and Dissemination in York
- MEDLINE
- Embase
- Specialised databases available on the Web
- The National Research Register.

Resources

To access these databases the public health professional who is expected to manage evidence requires a computer with a modem, a subscription to a provider with a link to the Internet, a software browser, and conversions management software.

Perhaps, most important of all, they require access to the skills of a librarian who must be fully competent in the field of electronic as opposed to paper information, for it is the librarian who will have to help the public health professional develop the skills they need to find, appraise, store and use information in those times when information is needed but a librarian is not available. Evenings and weekends are often times when evidence has to be gathered for decision-making.

The Chief Knowledge Officer

It is said that some American private companies are now appointing or designating a Chief Knowledge Officer, a board-level player of equivalent status to the other chief officers of the company and directly accountable to the Chief Executive. The job of the Chief Knowledge Officer is to manage the knowledge in the organisation, to pick up new knowledge and make sure that the organisation is acting upon it, and to develop systems for managing knowledge.

The Director of Public Health should be the Chief Knowledge Officer of a health authority; but how well do we manage knowledge within departments of public health? What decision has the department made, for example, about the balance that should be struck between searching and scanning in the allocation of time, and therefore resources, in the department? Within scanning, whether three journals are scanned or 30, how is responsibility for scanning allocated and how are the important papers found by scanning related to the work of the department, and therefore the authority? The development of systems for managing knowledge are necessary for every organisation but are particularly important for those departments which claim to be the best at managing knowledge and who have a lead for this function within the organisation.

The future of evidence-based decision-making

One of the main benefits of the campaign to promote evidence-based decision-making, and campaign is an appropriate metaphor, has been that it has clarified the different types of propositions that make up a decision.

In the past, decision-making involved a welter of propositions, none of which were clearly categorised or distinguished in type, with the exception of obvious statements of prejudice such as a racist or sexist remark, although these too were often overlooked. The focus on evidence-based decision-making has led to the distinction between:

- propositions supported by research evidence
- propositions based on personal experience
- propositions based on values
- propositions relating to resources.

This distinction has been helpful and it is unlikely that people will revert to a style of decision-making in which these types of categories or propositions are not distinguished and not appreciated during the course of the decision-making.

It is, however, appropriate to look into the future and to ask whether this style of decision-making will be universally acceptable and gain increasing, or decreasing, influence. At the heart of this, particularly in clinical practice, lies the management of uncertainty. In the Editor's column in the *British Medical Journal* of 6 May 1999, the Editor quoted Dr David Pencheon as saying that the three most important words in the clinician's vocabulary were 'I don't know', and that the whole future of education should be based on a different paradigm from that which expected every clinician to know everything. This approach – rooted in evidence-based decision-making that emphasises the importance of asking the right question, finding the best evidence, and appraising it critically – brings uncertainty to the forefront of decision-making. This is not, however, what people always want when they are anxious. In parallel with the development of evidence-based decision-making and the celebration of uncertainty is the rapid expansion of complementary and alternative therapies in which uncertainty is not even hinted at. Thus we may see in the future an inexorable move towards evidence-based decision-making among the clinicians and managers with an inexorable trend towards dissatisfaction with health care and clinical practice and a search for alternatives which are based on certainty among a large, and perhaps increasing, number of patients. Thus, the future of evidence-based decision-making may be intimately interwoven with the growth of medical fundamentalism.

References

Department of Health (1998) *Information for Health: An Information Strategy for the Modern NHS*. DoH, Wetherby.

Eddy D.M. (1993) Three battles to watch in the 1990s. *Journal of the American Medical Association*, **270**, 520–26.

Fullard E., Fowler G. & Gray J.A.M. (1984) Facilitating prevention in primary care. *British Medical Journal*, **289**, 1585–7.

Gray J.A.M. (1997) *Evidence-Based Healthcare*. Churchill Livingstone, London.

Halberstam D. (1972) *The Best and the Brightest*. Random House, New York.

Hope T. (1996) *Evidence-Based Patient Choice*. King's Fund Publishing, London.

House of Lords Select Committee on Science and Technology (1987–88) *Priorities in Medical Research*. House of Lords Session 1987–88, **54**. HMSO, London.

Sackett D.L., Haynes R.B. & Tugwell P. (1985) *Clinical Epidemiology: a Basic Science for Clinical Medicine*. Little, Brown and Company, Boston.

Sackett D.L., Haynes B.L., Guyatt G.H. & Tugwell P. (1991) *Clinical Epidemiology: a Basic Science for Clinical Medicine* (2nd edition). Little, Brown and Company, Boston.

Sackett D.L., Richardson W.S., Rosenberg W. & Haynes R.B. (1997) *Evidence-Based Medicine: How to Practise and Teach EBM*. Churchill Livingstone, London.

Sackett D.L., Rosenberg W.M.C., Gray J.A.M., Haynes R.B. & Richardson W.S. (1996) Evidence-based medicine: what it is and what it isn't. British Medical Journal, **312**, 71–2.

Spengler O. (1991) *The Decline of the West*. Oxford University Press, Oxford.

Chapter 6

Evidence-Based Nursing Practice

Richard Blomfield and Sally Hardy

Introduction

Nursing as a recognised occupation did not come into existence until the seventeenth century. Today, nurses make up nearly 70% of the National Health Service (NHS) workforce (Open College 1996). Despite this, the identity of nursing remains problematic. The knowledge, skills and values of nursing, midwifery and health visiting are all influenced by the wider economic, social and political contexts. Contemporary definitions of nursing, and of nursing research, are therefore bound in these contextual differences. Within this chapter the term 'nursing' is used as a shorthand to include all branches and specialties of nursing.

In the first section of this chapter an overview of the historical development of nursing as a profession is presented. The second section begins to explore the notion of evidence-based practice as a development within nursing. Finally, the debate moves to a critical consideration of the relevance of evidence-based practice for nursing and its place within contemporary health care. Evidence-based practice is in the early stages of development as we write, therefore our aim is to discuss critically and explore avenues of potential development, rather than present a completed picture of what the future holds for evidence-based nursing.

Recent developments in the organisation of the NHS require nursing to develop an identity based upon a solid understanding of its position within a health service which is 'modern and dependable' (Department of Health 1997). Little space (or courage) exists within the current culture to allow nursing the luxury of debate and exploration of uncertainty, yet we hope this chapter will trigger some nurses to enquire further into the appropriate evidence for their contemporary practice.

The professional development of nursing

Nursing is central to effective health care delivery. Studies in the USA are beginning to show that patient satisfaction increases and mortality rates are reduced within hospitals which ascribe high value to their nursing staff (Lancaster 1998). According to Professor Aiken, Director of the Centre for Health Services and Policy Research at the University of Pennsylvania, Philadelphia:

'it is the knowledge and judgement of nurses in direct patient care roles that will create the most affective healthcare organisations ... There is no managerial substitute for an expert nurse clinician's judgement'.

(Lancaster 1998)

Despite this, however, the history of nursing as a profession is one that has been characterised by difficulties in defining and asserting a distinctive professional identity. From within the profession there has been a long-standing tension between those who emphasise the technical and science-based aspects of nursing and those who emphasise the caring aspects of nursing. Allied to this has been what Perry (1993) terms the 'handmaiden' role of nursing, where the profession has developed in a continuously subservient role, directed by external forces. Nursing practice has evolved in the shadow of Victorian patriarchy, tainted as women's work, of low status, with poor pay and conditions, and with nurses working under, rather than alongside the medical profession (Oakley 1984). Throughout history, nursing has been and remains dominated by women. According to Delmothe (1988) the notion of nursing as 'women's work' has hindered any attempt to raise its professional status within society and in the eyes of the medical profession.

Although attempts have been made to define nursing in its many guises, very few can assert with confidence what a nurse is, or should be (Nightingale 1859; Henderson 1966; Peplau 1961; Roper *et al.* 1981; Roy 1981; Porter 1994; Hardy & Hally 1998) (see also Box 6.1).

As can be seen from Box 6.1, nursing is concerned broadly with restoring, maximising and maintaining the health and well-being of patients. What also appears important is that the broad range of nurses' roles and responsibilities be centred within the context of a constructive relationship between the nurse and the patient/client. The considerable variation in definitions presented in Box 6.1 does, however, highlight the enormous struggle and change which has occurred in both the professional and political contexts within which nursing has developed. Throughout history, nursing has had to respond to the changing demands of society and its health needs. It is also evident that key nursing commentators have themselves differed, with varying emphases on technical skill and compassion, science and art. Evidence-based nursing has emerged at a time when these divisions are accentuated in the clinical and educational setting.

> **Box 6.1: Definitions of nursing**
>
> *Nightingale (1881):* 'We want gentle women who come with settled purpose to do their work, free from all romance and affectation, but yet not wanting in some genuine enthusiasm.'
>
> *Peplau (1952):* defined nursing as therapeutic. 'It is a healing art, assisting an individual who is sick or in need of health care. Nursing can be viewed as an interpersonal process because it involves interaction between two people with a common goal.'
>
> *Orem (1959–1980):* defined nursing as having as its 'special concern the individual's needs for self-care action and provision and management of it, on a continuous basis in order to sustain life and health, recover from disease or injury and cope with the effects'.
>
> *Weidenbach (1964):* offers another slant in that, 'nursing is about nurturing and caring for someone in a motherly fashion. That care is given in the immediate present and can be given by any caring person. Nursing is a helping service that is rendered with compassion, skill and understanding of those who need care.'
>
> *Newman (1979):* views nursing as 'a unique profession that concerns itself with all the variables affecting human response to stressors, with primary concern for the total person. The primary goal of nursing is the retention and attainment of the clients' system stability.'

Early developments

It is difficult to explore the history of nursing without focusing on Florence Nightingale, although there have been other famous nurses before and after her (e.g. Elizabeth Fry, Louisa Twinning, Mary Seacole, Edith Cavell, Mrs Bedford Fenwick). However, it was Florence Nightingale's work in the Crimean War that altered the organisation and perception of nursing care. Her application of knowledge in the areas of sanitation, statistics, nutrition and public health affected not only the delivery and training of nursing but also affected social welfare. It has been argued that if Florence Nightingale encouraged nurses to practice as she did, the profession would be very different today. In reality, most of her effort was concerned with the organisation of the profession rather than encouraging the scrutiny and analysis of nursing work (Clifford 1990).

Nightingale opposed the registration of nurses. Her concern was not only for technical skills training but centred on attitude and personal character training. She argued strongly against a national register, as she believed this would be asking her nurses to perform an examination, and hence reduce them to 'dictionaries'. She was also concerned that national standards would have to be minimal standards, and that professional competence could not be judged on a single day and therefore not guaranteed beyond registration.

The two world wars added a further entry gate to nursing with the introduction of Red Cross Voluntary Aid Despatchment nurses who quickly proved they were able to work closely with patients and improve standards of care, albeit with minimal training. This challenged the assumption, established by Nightingale, that all nurses needed a three-year training.

In the post-war period the focus of nursing history shifted to America, from where practice and theory innovations and nursing research infiltrated back into Britain and Europe (Dingwall *et al.* 1986; Kelly & Joel 1996; Cormack 1996). According to Salvage (1998), this was not surprising as nursing lacked the basic infrastructure and culture of evaluation, which still remains limited today throughout Europe.

Contemporary practice

To this day the precise nature of nursing remains contested, with nursing subject, as ever, to contradictory forces, much of which remain outside of the profession's control. In the 1970s, the Briggs Report (DHSS 1972) called for nursing to be a research-based profession. The report prompted the most radical shake-up of nursing education since Nightingale, whereby nursing education was taken from the hospital setting and plans developed to merge nurse training with higher education. Project 2000 subsequently emerged in 1984, offering student nurses very different methods and means of training. What has arguably emerged from this is a rapid expansion and uptake within nursing of all aspects of research culture.

More recently, however, the Labour government in Britain, under Health Secretary Frank Dobson, has introduced further changes. These include significant alterations to the statutory professional bodies, including the abolition of separate national boards and the UKCC (the UK Central Council for Nursing, Midwifery and Health Visiting). As a response to the shortage of new recruits and the suboptimal retention of existing staff nurses in practice, the government also insisted that nurse training should place *less* emphasis on academic education, and more on practical training. At the same time, the introduction of PREP (the UKCC's post-registration and practice requirements) was an attempt to encourage nurses to be life-long learners.

As the new millennium dawns, nursing remains dogged by concerns over poor wages (Brindle 1998), working conditions, social standing and career development. The registration of nurses remains an unresolved issue. The continual need for updating, monitoring and registration of practice continues.

The organisational context

From the inception of the NHS in 1948, demand has outstripped the allotted and available financial resources (Salter 1998). Today the combination of an ageing, longer-living population, rising patient expectations, technological advances and the globalisation of health care information, has created a growing emphasis on cost-effectiveness to offset the burgeoning financial burden. This in turn has the knock-on effect of altering and challenging the preparation of nursing to meet the demands of contemporary health care. The document, *Vision for the Future* (HMSO 1993), summarises many of the major structural and managerial changes introduced within health care in the UK (Box 6.2).

Box 6.2: Contemporary health care changes

Influential changes to health care provision:

(1) Increased professional responsibility for nurses to take more active role in health promotion.

(2) Expansion of highly technical and expensive therapeutic approaches in health care treatments.

(3) Increased public awareness, information access and expectations of services.

(4) An increased longevity within the population.

(5) Health care decentralised and provided by a number of different agencies.

(6) Increased patient throughput, turnover and expectations.

(7) Emphasis on care in the community and the closing of large institutions.

(8) Restriction on funding and resources, with an emphasis on efficiency, effectiveness and value for money.

Solutions to these problems are being actively sought through a health service that has:

- a preoccupation with cost control
- developed systems to prevent costs falling on the individual
- increasing emphasis on purchasing health care
- increasing public and political interest in the evidence on which decisions about the effectiveness and safety of health care interventions are made.

One significant response to these challenges in the UK has been the introduction of the clinical governance initiative (Department of Health 1998). Whilst traditionally health care managers have left almost all clinical decision-making to the clinicians themselves (Salter 1998), the introduction of the clinical governance initiative has unsettled the previous balance of accountability and power. Chief executives are now ultimately accountable for the care of the patients within their trusts. This emphasis on account-ability has led to the need for highly visible, well-researched guidelines for practitioners to follow. It has been suggested that there will be some 50 guidelines each year over the 10-year strategy for improvement and modernisation of the NHS. In 1999, the National Institute for Clinical Excellence (NICE) was established with the main aim of producing and disseminating clinical guidelines (Department of Health 1997). Baroness Jay, in her role as Minister for Health, states:

> 'we support the regulation of professionals by professionals. Clinical governance builds on this. But we also want the professionals and others to consider how self-regulation might be strengthened and modernised so that it remains open and accountable to public scrutiny and responsive to changing clinical practice and service need'.
>
> (Jay 1998)

Clinical governance will affect all nurses whether they work in the community, in hospitals or on trust boards. The current momentum towards clinical governance presents nursing with a significant window of opportunity. *The New NHS, modern, dependable* (Department of Health 1997), if fully implemented, could lead to major changes in the division of labour within the NHS, a redefinition of some key tasks and even the redistribution of power (Klein 1998). Corresponding White Papers for Wales, Scotland and Northern Ireland will have a similar effect.

Klein (1998) argues that if nurses are to grasp the opportunities presented by this White Paper they need to develop new ways of defining nursing. This would enable nurses to manage the interface between health care and the wider community. The most important challenge is for nurses to achieve a strong representation on the proposed NICE, since this will help define the currency of accountability in the NHS (Klein 1998). In order to do so, however, nursing will have to move beyond its traditional handmaiden role.

The research background

Some of the uncertainties and tensions evident in the professional development of nursing are played out in the profession's relationship with research. There has been an enormous increase in the number of nurse researchers, academics and nursing journals over the past two decades. Many new journals have been established to accommodate the debates and processes that nursing research is bringing to the surface. Yet the impact of nursing research has been hampered by two problems. First, nursing is a relative newcomer to the research world, and has struggled to establish and assert its distinctive voice; second, like many other professions, the relationship between research and actual practice is problematic.

Polit & Hungler (1991) provide a useful breakdown of different eras of nursing research over the decades. Research carried out in the 1940s and 1950s mostly focused on the training or work environment of nurses, whilst in the 1960s and 1970s the major concern of researchers was the development of nursing theories. These theorists have subsequently been criticised for gathering material from other disciplines, rather than concentrating on what was essentially nursing knowledge. It was not until the 1980s and 1990s that nursing research in Britain turned its attentions to a systematic enquiry into actual nursing practice, following an earlier movement in the US.

Hockey (1996) declares that research is by intent concerned with creating new knowledge through the process of systematic enquiry governed by scientific principles (Box 6.3). She defines nursing research as any research activity that predominantly and appropriately falls within the domain of nursing. Yet, as we have seen, exactly what does fall into the domain of nursing often remains unclear.

Box 6.3: Aims of nursing research

(1)   To establish scientifically defensible reasons for activities.

(2)   To provide an increased repertoire of scientifically defensible intervention options.

(3)   To increase the cost-effectiveness of activities.

(4)   To provide a basis for standard setting and quality assurance.

(5)   To provide evidence of weaknesses and strengths.

(6)   To provide evidence in support for demands for resources.

(7)   To satisfy academic curiosity.

(8)   To facilitate interdisciplinary collaboration.

(9)   To earn and defend a professional status.

Hockey 1996

Following the Briggs Report, there is an expectation that all nurses should be at least aware of the research process (Buckledee & Macmahon 1994). Research methods teaching is a compulsory part of all student nurse training. Both pre- and post-registration courses are being run to help nurses understand the research process, but it remains untested how far this is affecting clinical practice. Indeed, in a study carried out by Walsh & Ford (1989), many nursing activities were observed to be practised from a traditional 'we've always done it like this' stance rather than based on research findings. They argued that most of the day-to-day activities of nursing practice were rooted in myth and derived through ritualistic exercises. Tiernay (1996) declared that if the same study were to be carried out again today, inevitably practices that fly in the face of research evidence would be paramount.

Studies have identified that there are significant barriers to the uptake of research in pursuit of practice developments (Hunt 1981, 1996; Closs & Cheater 1994). A number of reasons have also been proposed for the failure of nurses to maintain, and implement up-to-date knowledge (Hunt 1996; RCN 1998; Thompson 1998; Walsh 1997; see also Box 6.4).

Box 6.4: Barriers to implementing new knowledge

- Lack of awareness of new evidence
- An absence of relevant and/or high-quality research
- Lack of resources, e.g. journals, databases, libraries
- Limited time restricts the ability or motivation to find or implement new evidence
- Lack of expertise in the appraisal of research quality, power and relevance
- Reliance on out-of-date information from text books, colleagues or original training programme
- Anxiety over the idea of changing practice, possibly due to resistance within the working environment.

Some writers are therefore beginning to emphasise the need for appropriate strategies for the promotion of a new set of skills for clinical nurses, and a greater coordination of information (McMahon & Kitson 1997). The current literature also explores whether nursing lacks the infrastructure to promote scholastic research and evidence-based practice (McKenna & Mason 1998; Curzio 1998).

The emergence of evidence-based nursing

At present clinical decision-making in nursing (an area currently under investigation by the English National Board for Nursing, Midwifery and health visiting) is based upon one or more of the following:

(1) Clinical experience
(2) Observation
(3) Training
(4) Classroom and/or peer group teaching
(5) Written and published material
(6) Personal and/or team-based research.

As an individual process, such decision-making is now being challenged through the emergence of evidence-based practice, as well as through clinical governance.

Gray (1997) describes evidence-based health care as a discipline centred upon evidence-based decision-making about individual patients, groups of patients or populations, which may manifest as evidence-based purchasing or evidence-based management. Evidence-based clinical practice is further defined as an approach to decision-making in which the clinician uses the best evidence available, in consultation, to decide upon the option which best suits the patient (Gray 1997). Even where evidence is hard to find, the practitioner is still expected to find and assess what evidence there is, appraise it, utilise it and evaluate its use. There is increasing pressure to base clinical decisions on evidence and not on personal opinion-based judgements. The health care decision-maker of the twenty-first century will be expected to make decisions about clinical practice based upon a systematic appraisal of the best evidence available relating to that decision (Gray 1997).

The skills required for evidence-based decision-making are as follows:

- the ability to define criteria such as effectiveness, safety, and acceptability
- the ability to find articles on effectiveness, safety and the acceptability of new treatments
- the ability to assess the quality of the evidence
- the ability to assess whether the results of the research are generalisable
- the ability to assess whether the results of the research are applicable to the local population (i.e. case load or client group).

Evidence-based nursing initiatives

The rapid move towards evidence-based practice throughout the health field is beginning to find echoes from within nursing. Over the last few years a number of evidence-based nursing initiatives have been established. These initiatives mirror developments in evidence-based medicine in three ways. The first point of similarity is the shared definition of evidence-based practice which underpins initiatives in nursing and medicine. Thus DiCenso *et al.* (1998) define evidence-based nursing as:

> 'The process by which nurses make clinical decisions using the best available research evidence, their clinical expertise and patient preferences, in the context of available resources'.
>
> DiCenso *et al.* (1998)

This definition has considerable parallels with that proposed for evidence-based medicine by Sackett *et al.* (1996).

The second point of similarity is that the aims of the initiatives set up in nursing mirror those of wider, evidence-based health initiatives, by focusing on the key processes within evidence-based practice: generating evidence, appraising and disseminating evidence, and providing training on identifying, appraising and using evidence. Finally, it is worth noting that the impetus for initiatives has frequently come from enthusiasts within the profession, rather than under the lead of the major professional bodies. Some of the more important initiatives are highlighted below.

Evidence-based nursing centres

The Centre for Evidence-Based Nursing (CEBN) at the University of York focuses on developing evidence-based nursing through education, research and development. Research activities in the centre include:

(1) Generating evidence through primary research and systematic review, with projects including systematic reviews of wound care (through the Cochrane Wounds Group) and a multicentre RCT (randomed controlled trial) of compression bandages for people with leg ulcers.
(2) Research on nurses' use of research information in decision-making.
(3) Evaluation of the impact of teaching evidence-based nursing on clinical practice and organisations.

The Centre for Evidence-Based Practice, located in the Wolfson Institute of Health Sciences, Thames Valley University, also aims to develop evidence-based nursing through undertaking research and the dissemination of research findings to practitioners. The centre is currently involved in an RCT of strategies for reducing crying and sleeping problems in newborn babies, as well as a study to evaluate a strategy of using research to improve care of patients with leg ulcers.

The Joanna Briggs Institute for Evidence-Based Nursing and Midwifery is a multicentre collaboration of supporting centres in Australia, Hong Kong and New Zealand (http://www.joannabriggs.edu.au/). The aims of the institute are to:

(1) Identify areas where nurses and other health professionals most urgently require summarised evidence.
(2) Carry out and facilitate systematic reviews of international research.
(3) Undertake multi-site randomised controlled clinical trials in areas where good evidence is not available.
(4) Prepare easy-to-read summaries of best practice in the form of practice information sheets, based on the results of systematic reviews.
(5) Design and conduct targeted dissemination activities in areas where (or when) good evidence is available.

Information services

The Nursing and Midwifery Audit Information Service, funded by the UK Department of Health, with the support of the Royal College of Nursing, provides help with locating evidence and guidelines, drawing particularly on work done by the NHS Centre for Reviews and Dissemination and the Cochrane Collaboration.

The Network for Psychiatric Nursing Research (NPNR) is a UK-based service launched in 1996, funded by the Department of Health and located in Oxford. It provides a search and information service for health professionals in mental health nursing, and publishes a regular newsletter called *NetLink*.

Journals

The international journal *Evidence-Based Nursing* is published quarterly, and was started in January 1998 as a joint venture of the BMJ Publishing Group and Royal College of Nursing. It joins a stable of similar publications, including *Evidence-Based Medicine* and *Evidence-Based Mental Health*. The journal publishes structured summaries of quantitative and qualitative research relating to nursing accompanied by a 'value-added' summary of the clinical applications of the article. The journal has developed specific criteria for selecting, evaluating and abstracting quantitative and qualitative studies.

Early indications are that there is a fair amount of interest in evidence-based practice among nurses. The journal *Evidence-Based Nursing* has rapidly built up a large number of subscribers. The Royal College of Nursing publication *Update* (1998) on clinical effectiveness offers guidelines on how to find and appraise evidence. This information gives nurses some ideas on how evidence-based nursing practice and effective clinical decision-making can work in practice settings. Many other illustrations of actual practice examples are quickly filtering through (McClarey & Duff 1997; Thompson 1998; McInnes *et al.* 1998; Sullivan 1998).

A glance at the journal *Evidence-Based Nursing* indicates the wealth of research evidence that nurses from around the world have produced. Valuable discoveries are being made and the knowledge base on which nursing can draw is growing at an exponential rate. The areas of nursing under examination are extremely diverse. For example, the January 1999 (Vol. 2 No. 1) edition of *Evidence-Based Nursing* included the following:

- venipuncture was less painful and more efficient than heel lance for blood testing in newborns
- skills training reduced sexual risk behaviours in homeless men with mental illness

- early discharge after surgery for breast cancer was safe and well received by patients
- obese binge-eating women had no weight loss with diet or non-diet therapies
- integration of services for elderly people reduced cost and use of health services
- nurse-led secondary prevention clinics improved health and decreased hospital admissions in patients with coronary heart disease
- regular exercise during pregnancy did not affect physical growth or mental development of infants
- therapeutic communities helped people to recover from substance abuse and implement new lives.

The following section considers whether the new-found enthusiasm for evidence-based practice represents a positive or negative development for nursing.

The potential and pitfalls of evidence-based nursing

The essential value of evidence-based practice is the emphasis it places on rational action through a structured appraisal of empirical evidence, rather than the adherence to blind conjecture, dogmatic ritual or private intuition. Its value for the delivery of effective health care interventions is unquestionable. As an axiomatic statement of rational behaviour the idea is hardly worthy of discussion.

Across a range of professions, it has been evident that the influence of research on practice has been limited, with practitioners rarely altering their practice on the basis of research findings (Bergin & Strupp 1972). The experimental approach of RCTs with large sample groups offers the promise that a certain treatment will be of general use, even to individual patients with their very complex human problems (Barlow *et al.* 1984). Furthermore, in the past, closer examination of new procedures has often revealed that their popularity had more to do with effective communication and workshops to influence change rather than evidence of convincing data. For example cognitive therapy, developed and popularised by Beck, was widely adopted and regarded as an effective time-limited therapy before any convincing data was available on the effectiveness of the procedure within a clinical population (Barlow *et al.* 1984: 36). The growth of a truly evidence-based culture in health care may help to guard against this type of over-enthusiastic response in the future.

The growth of a cross-disciplinary movement towards evidence-based practice is also to be welcomed. It is important to realise that not all studies that come under the banner of evidence-based nursing, and included in the journal of that name, are nurse-designed or nurse-led. Indeed the collaborative nature of much of the emerging work is a sign of the way the evidence-based practice movement may have an important role for the sharing or cross-pollination of knowledge between disciplines.

Finally, the emphasis on accountability, quality and efficiency of health care within both clinical governance and evidence-based practice is long overdue. It is true of human nature that people tend to take more responsibility for their actions if they know they may be called to account to a higher authority.

Nonetheless, we do have significant reservations about the development of evidence-based practice, and evidence-based nursing in particular. Reflecting on nursing's past to present-day developments pose many questions about the introduction of evidence-based practice. The central questions are:

(1) Does evidence-based practice lead to greater professional autonomy for nursing?
(2) Does evidence-based practice improve patient care?
(3) Will evidence-based practice empower consumers?
(4) What has nursing to gain from embracing evidence-based practice?
(5) Does nursing already practice evidence-based nursing in another guise?

Definitions of evidence

Those who have championed evidence-based medicine, also champion RCTs as the best evidence or the gold standard for judging the risks and benefits of treatments. It is notable that although some qualitative studies are used as evidence, and summarised in the journal *Evidence-Based Nursing* (see above under *Journals*, this chapter), those of a quantitative nature predominate. The overriding message, however, appears to be that quantitative research provides a stronger evidence base than interpretative, or qualitative, methods. This is even emphasised in symbolic form by the Cochrane Collaboration logo, which depicts the findings of RCTs. 'Soft' forms of research are frequently rated as having only limited value as research-based evidence (Royal College of Nursing 1998).

It could be argued that taking this polarised view of research methods, or narrow definition of what constitutes evidence, is problematic within the domain of nursing in a number of ways. Although nursing publications are awash with research and notions of evidence-based practice, nurses remain divided as to whether any of these articles relate to them. Perhaps the main reason why many nurses have so far failed to embrace evidence-based practice with enthusiasm is that it holds limited relevance for their everyday practice needs. Nurses do not operate in predictable, determinate conditions where they can adequately rely upon the narrow definition of 'evidence' found in evidence-based practice, synonymous with what Schon called 'technical rationality' (Schon 1983). Rather, they must respond to the challenges of messy 'indeterminate swamplands' (Schon 1983) in which unpredictable value conflicts reduce the traditional positivist approach to only marginal significance (Schon 1983). In such a context the confused practitioner can all too readily blame themselves for failure to implement research findings into practice (Hunt 1981; Gould 1986; Armitage 1991).

But, as Carper (1978, 1996) explains, this empirical knowledge is only one form of knowing. Carper describes three other interrelated patterns of knowing: personal, ethical and esthetic. The personal way of knowing refers to all that we understand in a private, untestable way. Its enhancement marks the transition from 'novice to expert' (Benner 1984). This is the human universe of the nurse as he or she struggles to make sense of complex practice situations and interpersonal relations. Here too, the nurse must draw on ethical knowledge in order to manage conflicts of values, and an esthetic ability to conceptually grasp complex situations in order to respond to them effectively.

Barlow *et al.* (1984) offer a warning to what they call 'crystal ball gazing' where practitioners become little more than technicians. The limitations of applying the findings of RCTs to individual patients/clients is often best understood by nurses who tend to see individuals more as whole beings rather than simply the sum of their parts. This has been partly reflected by the types of research which nurses have undertaken. Within the British context, a search of the Department of Health's *National Research Register* 1988 No. 1 issue indicates that the vast majority of research undertaken by nurses has a significant interpretative component. There are very few RCTs led by nurses.

For clinical nursing to progress, each practitioner needs to develop as an applied researcher, in that they seek the appropriate information to inform their judgement of care (Schostak 1998). Nurses risk becoming expert mimics if they take up the gauntlet of evidence-based practice without a critical mind. Relying on one source of evidence (for example, one RCT) is like watching black and white television. A core of information might be present, but in widescreen technicolour the impression may be totally different.

An anecdotal illustration

Several years ago, the *Guardian* newspaper's advertisement campaign showed a picture of a punk rocker walking along a busy street. He was approaching a man in a suit holding a briefcase. The punk rocker is seen looking at and making a grab for the suited man. Only when the picture scans back does the audience get to see the fuller picture. Overhead there is a large object falling off scaffolding. The punk rocker is in reality pushing the man out of harm rather than making a grab for his briefcase. Without the full picture, evidence-based nursing practice will merely act as a reinforcer for many professional assumptions, leaving the new and sometimes unexpected evidence either unbelieved or unseen (Schratz & Walker 1995).

Furthermore, appraisal of systematic reviews is not at all easy or straightforward. It has to be conducted with common sense and vigilance, in that statistical data still need to be interpreted within the correct context. It is important not to lose sight of qualitative variables influencing the hard data (Kirkwood 1988).

The practice of evidence-based health care aims to enable those managing health services to determine the mix of services and procedures that will give the greatest benefit to the population it serves. However there is no guarantee that any potential benefits will be realised in practice. Outcome measures, for example, popular as a means of measuring success in modern health care, often fail to identify the context or individual complexities of procedures and are most often determined by the quality of the process. Quality management is therefore essential in supporting the clinicians to produce evidence-based practice, with low risk and reasonable cost, from the resources available.

If nurses are to have the confidence and self-esteem to work inter-dependently as key players within the multidisciplinary team they must come to accept that the realities of nursing cannot always be reduced to hard (i.e. measurable, observable, repeatable) data. To supplement and enhance the emerging evidence-based culture, nursing must draw upon, rather than abandon, the wealth of nursing theory which has developed exponentially over the last few decades (Chinn & Kramer 1991; Crossan & Robb 1998; Fraser 1996; Kikuchi & Simmons 1992; Kitson 1993; Marriner-Tomey 1994; McKenna & Mason 1997; Perry 1997; Wesley 1995). The complexities involved in the analysis of the conceptual and syntactical structure of nursing knowledge has long been understood by nurse theorists. Little known to the outside world, nurses have endeavoured to capture the essence of practice through an exploration of the epistemological underpinnings of nursing action.

Reflective practice and the theory–practice gap

The concept of reflective practice has been explored at length in the nursing literature. The work of Schon (1983) for example helped to illuminate the complexity of professional work. Central to his thesis was the idea that the traditional technical way of rationalising professional work was not appropriate since this failed to capture the complex nature of such work. He pointed to the importance of 'tacit' knowledge. Much of what a professional does, he argued, is a reflection of the conjunction between what the professional has learnt as theory, and what they have internalised through experience. He claimed that this 'knowledge-in-action' might be difficult if not impossible to articulate. Such knowledge, according to Schon, comes from two types of reflection: reflection-*in*-action; and reflection-*on*-action. The first occurs whilst the action is taking place, and the second, after the event.

Further exploration of the nature of reflective practice came about with the work of Kolb (1984), who described how the experiential learner could use reflection to conceptualise concrete experiences. Kolb and other authors (Boyd & Fales 1983; Boud *et al.* 1985) developed a working notion of reflective practice as a process in which the professional explores experience in order to bring about changes in understanding. Boud *et al.* (1985) gave the following definition:

'Reflection in the context of learning is a generic term for those intellectual and affective activities in which individuals engage to explore their experiences in order to lead to new understanding and appreciations'.

(Boud *et al.* 1985: 19)

There are many examples of the gulf between what is taught, and that which is done (Butterworth & Faugier 1992). Some authors argue that, rather than presenting us with a problem, the apparent dichotomy between theory and practice actually stimulates reflective learning by setting up a dynamic tension, the resolution of which constitutes informed action, or praxis (Argyris & Schon 1974; Cox *et al.* 1991; Johns 1995). In transcending the contradictions between theory and practice, a dialectic process leads us to a creative synergy.

Benner (1984) states that:

'A further value of reflective practice is its natural phenomenological focus on lived experience. With guidance it offers a collaborative research approach to work with practitioners and students to research their lived experiences of practice towards developing nursing knowledge embedded in everyday practitioners' experiences.'

(Benner 1984)

Here we have a clear appreciation of what Kikuchi (1992) described as 'private ways of knowing'. Although such knowledge may be 'incommunicable and publicly unverifiable' it may nevertheless make up a large part of what the practising nurse actually knows. The nurse is encouraged to move along the 'passage from detached observer, standing outside the situation, to one of a position of involvement, fully engaged in the situation' (Benner *et al.* 1992). Moving from the passive to the proactive approach means the nurse takes full responsibility for their actions. They become the creators of practice rather than the unwilling victims. These qualities are central to practice today, where nurses stand accountable for their own actions (UKCC 1992a). It also means that as a self-regulating practitioner, the nurse is able to expand, enhance and monitor their own practice (UKCC 1992b), without the need for continual prompting from others. This kind of self-regulation is a central characteristic of professional behaviour and a key requirement of the clinical governance iniative.

Of course, these ideals will only be achieved to the degree that the working environment nurtures and encourages a reflective approach. A judgmental, oppressive, rule-based environment will inhibit the development of reflective skills (Clarke *et al.* 1996). The 'life-strategy of communion' is characterised by an open, sharing attitude, with a readiness to accept new ideas. The natural consequence does seem to be that, through a reflective approach to practice, nurses come to care for the person and not the disease, the whole, and not simply the parts.

Embrace or abandon? Nursing's dilemma

We noted above how vulnerable nursing has been to definition from outside of the profession, from government and from other more powerful professions, especially medicine. The rapid development of evidence-based practice within the field of health and the associated concept of clinical governance, has posed something of a dilemma for nursing. In many senses evidence-based practice and clinical governance represent further externally imposed changes on nursing.

The development of clinical governance does have the effect of shifting responsibility for delivery of an appropriate, effective, efficient and economic service away from central government, thereby enhancing professional autonomy; but at the same time the profession is simultaneously placed in the position of being effectively policed from outside. Tattam & Thompson (1993: 127–8) poignantly remind us that:

'politicians use the NHS and nurses as the caring face of the service to score political points, but few are able to grasp its complexities ... it is important to remember that in politics it is the present that counts above all else, nurses have had to learn this the hard way'.

This does not mean however that everything originating from the government think-tanks should be treated with cynicism or resistance. Rather, nursing must creatively explore and expound the true implications and possibilities of each consultation paper (Thomas 1998). The notion of evidence-based practice is no exception to that rule. When the emergence of evidence-based practice is viewed as the offspring of the politicisation of health care (Salter 1998) the response of nurses may take on a rather more complex character.

Although there have been advances in the establishment of nursing as a research-based profession, many nurses find it hard to engage with research in their own areas. Many view evidence-based practice with scepticism and the dilemma facing them is whether to embrace, or effectively abandon the requirements of evidence-based practice. The reason why some government policies fail to capture the imagination of health professionals is that they are seen as mind-numbingly irrelevant to the realities of health provision. Hidden agendas generally become transparent once the professions have extracted the truth from the jargon (Jolley & Brykczyñska 1993). This mistrust and perceived lack of ownership of new ideas (such as evidence-based practice and clinical governance) may partially explain the notorious inertia with which individual nurses have traditionally adopted them.

With evidence-based practice the dilemma becomes even more apparent in the light of our discussion above about the restricted view of nursing, and the nurse–patient relationship, offered by evidence-based practice. There are real dangers for nursing if it unquestioningly adopts the medical-model definition of evidence-based practice, a problem evident in previous attempts to raise the status of the profession:

> 'Nursing, in its pursuit of technical knowledge, has tended to denigrate the value of caring skills ... the reasons why nurses have not valued caring skills can be viewed as the behaviour of an oppressed group striving to internalize the norms of the dominant group in a (false) belief that they will become more like the dominant group with increased status and recognition'.
>
> (Johns 1995)

On the other hand the profession may have little choice other than to adopt evidence-based practice or risk being left behind other health professions. More positively stated, evidence-based practice does offer significant advantages which the profession should willingly embrace. In order to do so, however, evidence-based nursing requires a broader definition of evidence.

The contribution of interpretative research

We have so far proposed that as much learning takes place in the unique, uncertain and complex situations of the 'swampy lowlands' of clinical practice, as does on the 'high hard ground' of fact-based learning (Schon 1991). This development in perspective cannot be over-emphasised since it represents the acknowledgement of the rich artistry of nursing, and hence opens the doors to a whole new genre of nursing research. The last two decades have seen the adoption of interpretative methodologies which were previously the domain of other better established social sciences

(Burns & Grove 1987; Holm 1997; Johnson & Webb 1995; LoBiondo-Wood & Haber 1998; Meyer 1993; Nichols 1997).

Interpretative research comes in many guises (Holm 1997). Nursing has made significant departures from the traditional methods of the natural sciences through the adoption of interpretative methodologies such as action research, grounded theory, ethnography and phenomenology. Exploring the complexity of human life lends itself well to both inter-pretative and quantitative exploration. Developing coherent arguments, deduced from empirical observations that recognise the dynamic pro-cesses, symbolic meanings and multivariate relations of nursing practice, is the most appropriate way of constructing an explanation of complex phenomena (Alford 1998: 19). Cross-sectional and interpretative methods have proven most useful in many other behavioural sciences and may provide more appropriate evidence (Risdale 1995).

Until recently, the social sciences have been intimidated by the sup-remacy claimed by positivistic approaches (Polkingthorne 1983). Yet the limitations of the *natural* sciences were highlighted in the nineteenth cen-tury by the German philosopher Wilhelm Dilthey (Mitchell & Cody 1996). Dilthey viewed the dominant methods of the natural sciences as 'a sterile empiricism that disconnected life from knowledge, [which] stripped life of human meaning and purpose' (Mitchell & Cody 1996). He proposed that only *human* science could truly aid our quest to understand persons, and that this would require concepts, theories and methods that were funda-mentally different from those used by the natural sciences. The main concern of the latter is the induction of physical laws through a process of conjecture and experimental observation leading to corroboration or refutation (Popper 1959). Human science, however, is concerned with the values and meaning of lived experiences, 'the interrelation of life, expression, and understanding' (Dilthey 1976: 175).

More recently the nursing literature has echoed Dilthey's concerns over the domination of the scientific method in health research (Gorenberg 1983; Munhall 1982; Newman 1979; Smith 1984; Vredevoe 1984; Webster *et al.* 1981).

The critical point is this: if the adoption of evidence-based practice means that nurses must disregard all but the most rigorous of scientific data, there is little wonder that many approach the process with a profound inertia. The future of evidence-based practice might depend on whether the notion of evidence is flexible enough to form a coherent part of the nursing universe.

In reality, our knowledge can never be free from interpretative elements. Of all the myths surrounding the traditional scientific endeavour, the myth of objectivity ranks amongst the most insidious (Chinn 1996). Even the most influential philosophers of science have shown that science can never guarantee the truth of its conclusions (Popper 1959; Kuhn 1970; Lakatos

1970) – nevertheless the myth lives on. Even those who pride themselves on the rigour of their scientific approach retain elements of interpretation in the traditional discussion section of their papers (Holm 1997).

In contrast, phenomenology (of the Heideggerian method) emphasises the pre-understanding (i.e. bias and prejudice) of the observer and rejects all notions of objective truth. These central methodological assumptions have been ultilised widely in nursing research. Unfortunately, it is unlikely that much of this research is generalisable in the way required by evidence-based nursing.

The emphasis on what is considered a strong method for evidence-based research does need to change. The large sample population studies that depersonalise patient groupings need not always be the best evidence. There is an ongoing move towards alternative research approaches and interest in individual patients observed within their particular environment (e.g. single-case methodology). Barlow *et al.* (1984) argue strongly that traditional scientific methodology alone is not always the most appropriate to answer major questions relevant to applied settings. An alternative scientific and empirical approach is needed.

The notion of client–treatment matching, or client–treatment interactions is one such approach (Garfield & Bergin 1978; Kendall & Butcher 1982). Barlow *et al.* (1984) also advocate time series methodology and clinical case replication. Time series is defined as a method that concentrates on monitoring change over a period of time alongside that of clinical replication where patients with the same problems are observed (over time), receive specific treatments and their reactions monitored. These approaches can offer the answer to important questions that large-scale studies fail to report.

The convergence of research strategies

An awareness of these limitations has led some to argue that interpretative methods of research differ from more traditional scientific methods solely to the extent that each employs an interpretative element (Holm 1997). They are commensurable since they essentially share the same paradigm (Holm 1997; Kuhn 1970). On the face of it, research using phenomenology or action research will appear very different from that using a strictly scientific methodology. Despite this 'there can be no doubt that some of the findings generated by qualitative research constitute knowledge in the commonly used sense of the word' (Holm 1997). Given all that has been said about the place held by interpretative forms of research within nursing, it would appear that the emerging culture of evidence-based practice must embrace a broader definition of evidence than is currently allowed, if it is to attain optimal relevance to the profession.

In recognition of this the journal *Evidence-Based Nursing* does include qualitative studies alongside quantitative studies. The journal is alone amongst its stable-mates, *Evidence-Based Medicine*, *ACP Journal Club* and *Evidence-Based Mental Health*, in currently including qualitative studies. Nonetheless, this attempt to broaden out the concept of evidence-based practice is in its early stages, and significant difficulties still require resolution.

The integration of qualitative or interpretative research into the evidence-based practice framework will not be straightforward. The sophisticated procedures developed for evidence-based practice have been designed with quantitative, especially RCT, research in mind. Even the most cursory reading of the qualitative summaries in *Evidence-Based Nursing* indicates that they fit rather uneasily within the format designed for very different research designs.

Qualitative research, designed to capture the complexity of experiences, perceptions and processes is not readily, even appropriately, reduced to a 450-word summary, nor is the sense of certainty conveyed by the term 'evidence' one with which many qualitative researchers will feel comfortable. Incorporating qualitative research may require considerable adaptation to the evidence-based practice model in order to avoid distorting qualitative research. Whether this is possible, or whether it would be welcomed by the architects of evidence-based practice, is an issue for further debate.

Conclusion: evidence of a future

> 'The philosophers have only interpreted the world in different ways; the point is to change it'.
>
> (Marx, 1844)

The real value of evidence-based practice actually lies in its cultural significance. As a statement of intent it has power to draw together the disparate elements of the various health care professions under the umbrella of a common goal. Its underlying philosophy and driving force is *collaborative pragmatism*, and this will require the end of isolationist practices in the field of health research.

If the goals of evidence-based practice are to be realised a multidisciplinary approach to change management is required. This is what sets evidence-based practice apart from other historical developments in nursing practice which have tended to be unidisciplinary in nature (Sleep 1998). A central feature of this culture is the imperative to forge partnerships with colleagues within the organisation whilst drawing on the expertise of external agencies including academic colleagues and the social, voluntary and commercial sectors (Sleep 1998; Wolfson Institute 1998).

New responsibilities create the need for new abilities, and the drive to make nursing an all-graduate profession was given strong support in a recent positional paper by the Council of Deans and Heads of University Faculties of Nursing, Midwifery and Health Visiting (Moore 1998). Furthermore, it is vital that nurses develop the skills and knowledge required to become respected partners in the commissioning of health care (Kaufman 1998). Basing practice on evidence gained from RCTs can undoubtedly be of great value to nursing practice. However, if the goals of evidence-based practice are to be realised *fully* by the nursing profession, the process must give more encouragement and recognition to eclectic, interpretative and novel/creative research methodologies. If these requirements were met, it would seem appropriate to predict that evidence-based practice will significantly affect the culture of health care provision in the twenty-first century.

References

Abbot P. & Sapsford R. (1992) *Research into Practice. A Reader for Nurses and Caring Professions*. Open University Press, Buckingham.

Abel-Smith B. (1960) *A History of the Nursing Profession*. Heinemann, London.

Alford R.R. (1998) *The Craft of Inquiry. Theories, Methods and Evidence*. Oxford University Press, Oxford.

Alavi C. (1995) *Problem-based Learning in a Health Sciences Curriculum*. Routledge, London.

Argyris C. & Schon D. (1974) *Theory in Practice: Increasing Professional Effectiveness*. Jossey-Bass, San Francisco.

Armitage S. (1991) Research utilisation in practice. *Nurse Education Today*, **10**, 10–15.

Barlow D.H., Hayes S.C. & Nelson R.O. (1984) *The Scientist Practitioner: Research and Accountability in Clinical and Educational Settings*. Allyn & Bacon, Massachusetts.

Benner P. (1984) *From Novice to Expert. Excellence and Power in Clinical Practice*. Addison Wesley, New York.

Benner P., Tanner C. & Chelsa C. (1992) From beginner to expert: Gaining a differentiated clinical world in critical care nursing. *Advances in Nursing Science*, **14**, 13–28.

Bergin A. & Strupp H. (1972) *Changing Frontiers in Science of Psychotherapy*. Aldine, Chicago.

Boud D., Keogh R. & Walker D. (1985) Promoting reflection in learning: a model. In D. Boud, R. Keogh & D. Walker (eds) *Reflection: Turning Experience into Learning*. Kogan Page, London.

Boyd E. & Fales A. (1983) Reflective learning: key to learning from experience. *Journal of Humanistic Psychology*, **23**, 99–117.

Briggs A. (1972) *Report of the Committee of Nursing*. HMSO, London.

Brindle D. (1998) Public sector pay awards: Nurses. *Guardian*, 30 January, p. 12.

Buckeldee J. & McMahon R. (1994) *The Research Experience in Nursing*. Chapman & Hall, London.

Burns N. & Grove S. (1987) *The Practice of Nursing Research* (3rd edition). W.B. Saunders Company, Philadelphia.

Butterworth T. & Faugier J. (eds) (1992) *Clinical Supervision and Mentorship in Nursing.* Chapman & Hall, London.

Carper B. (1978) Fundamental patterns of knowing in nursing. *Advances in Nursing Science,* **1**, 13–23.

Carper B. (1996) Fundamental patterns of knowing in nursing. In J. Kenney (ed.) *Philosophical and Theoretical Perspectives for Advanced Nursing Practice.* Jones and Bartlett, London.

Chinn P. (1996) Debunking myths in nursing theory and research. In J. Kenney (ed.) *Philosophical and Theoretical Perspectives for Advanced Nursing Practice.* Jones and Bartlett, London.

Chinn P. & Kramer M. (1991) *Theory and Nursing: a Systematic Approach* (3rd edn). Mosby Year Book, St Louis.

Clarke B., James C. & Kelly J. (1996) Reflective practice: reviewing the issues and refocusing the debate. *International Journal of Nursing Studies,* **33**, 171–80.

Clifford C. (1990) *Nursing and Health Care Research. A Skills-based Introduction* (2nd edn). Prentice Hall, Wiltshire.

Closs S.J. & Cheater F.M. (1994) Utilisation of nursing research: culture, interest and support. *Journal of Advanced Nursing,* **14**, 762–73.

Cormack D. (1996) *The Research Process in Nursing* (3rd edn). Blackwell Science Ltd, Oxford.

Cox H., Hickson P. & Taylor B. (1991) Exploring reflection: knowing and constructing practice. In G. Gray & R. Pratt (eds) *Towards a Discipline of Nursing.* Churchill Livingstone, Melbourne.

Crombie I., Davies H., Abrahma S. & Florey C. Du V. (1993) *The Audit Handbook. Improving Health Care Through Clinical Audit.* John Wiley & Sons, Chichester.

Crossan F. & Robb A. (1998) Role of the nurse: introducing theories and concepts. *British Journal of Nursing,* **7**, 608–12.

Curzio J. (1998) Funding for evidence-based nursing practice in the UK. *Nursing Times Research,* **3**, 100–107.

Delmothe T. (1988) Nursing grievances: voting with their feet. *British Medical Journal,* **296**, 25–8.

Department of Health (1996) *Clinical Effectiveness for the National Health Service.* HMSO, London.

Department of Health (1997) *The New NHS.* HMSO, London.

Department of Health (1998) *A First-Class Service: Quality in the New NHS.* HMSO, London.

DiCenso A., Cullum N. & Ciliska D. (1998) Implementing evidence-based nursing: some misconceptions [Editorial]. *Evidence-Based Nursing,* **1**, 38–40.

Dilthey W. (1976) *Selected Writings* (Rickman H., trans). Harper & Row, New York.

Dingwall R., Rafferty A. & Webster C. (1986) *An Introduction to the Social History of Nursing.* Routledge, London.

Docherty T. (ed.) (1993) *Postmodernism: A Reader.* Harvester Wheatsheaf, New York.

Donnison J. (1977) *Midwives and Medical Men. A History of Professional Rivalries and Women's Rights.* Heinemann, London.

Fraser M. (1996) *Conceptual Nursing Practice: A Research-Based Approach* (2nd edition). Chapman & Hall, London.

Garfield S. & Bergin A. (1978) *Handbook of Psychotherapy and Behaviour Change* (2nd edn). John Wiley, New York.

Goffman E. (1961) *Asylums. Essays on the Social Situation of Mental Patients and Other Inmates*. Penguin Books, Harmondsworth.

Gorenberg B. (1983) The research tradition of nursing: An emerging issue. *Nursing Research*, **32**, 347–9.

Gould D. (1986) Pressure sore prevention and treatment: an example of nurses' failure to implement research findings. *Journal of Advanced Nursing*, **11**, 389–94.

Gray J.M. (1997) *Evidence-based Healthcare*. Churchill Livingstone, Edinburgh.

Hardy S. & Hally H. (1998) Competent caring: roles of the mental health nurse. In B. Thomas, S. Hardy & P. Cutting (eds) *Stuart and Sundeen's Mental Health Nursing. Principles and Practice*. Mosby, London.

Henderson V. (1996) *The Nature of Nursing*. Macmillan, New York.

Hockey L. (1996) The nature and purpose of nursing research. In D. Cormack (ed.) *The Research Process in Nursing* (3rd edn). Blackwell Science, Oxford.

Holm S. (1997) The scientific status of qualitative research. In S. Holm (ed.) *Ethical Problems in Clinical Practice: the Ethical Reasoning of Health Care Professionals*. Manchester University Press, Manchester.

Hunt J. (1981) Indicators for nursing practice: the use of research findings. *Journal of Advanced Nursing*, **6**, 189–94.

Hunt J. (1996) Barriers to research utilisation. *Journal of Advanced Nursing*, **23**, 423–5.

Hyndman S. (1994) Leaping to the right conclusions? The problems of confounding variables and measurement in a ward-based nursing research project. In J. Buckledee & R. McMahon (eds) *The Research Experience in Nursing*. Chapman & Hall, London.

Jay (Baroness) (1998) Get in on the Act. *Nursing Standard*, **12** (43), 16.

Johns C. (1995) The value of reflective practice for nursing. *Journal of Clinical Nursing*, **4**, 23–30.

Johnson M. & Webb C. (1995) Rediscovering unpopular patients: the concept of social judgement. *Journal of Advanced Nursing*, **21**, 466–75.

Jolley M. (1993) Out of the Past. In M. Jolley & G. Brykczyñska (eds) *Nursing: its Hidden Agendas*. Edward Arnold, London.

Jolley M. & Brykczyñska G. (eds) (1993) *Nursing: its Hidden Agendas*. Edward Arnold, London.

Kaufman G. (1998) Commissioning: the community nurse's role. *Nursing Standard*, **12** (45), 35–7.

Kelly L. & Joel L. (1996) *The Nursing Experience. Trends, Challenges and Transitions* (3rd edn). McGraw Hill, New York.

Kendall P. & Butcher J. (1982) *Handbook of Research Methods in Clinical Psychology*. Wiley, New York.

Kikuchi J. (1992) Nursing questions that science cannot answer. In J.F. Kikuchi & H. Simmons (eds) *Philosophic Inquiry in Nursing*. Sage, London.

Kikuchi J. & Simmons H. (eds) (1992) *Philosophic Inquiry in Nursing*. Sage, London.

Kirkwood B. (1988) *Essentials of Medical Statistics*. Blackwell Science Publications, Oxford.

Kitson A. (ed.) (1993) *Nursing: Art and Science*. Chapman & Hall, London.

Klein R. (1998) Opportunity knocks ... will nurses answer? *Nursing Standard*, **12** (43), 26–7.

Kolb D. (1984) *Experiential Learning*. Prentice-Hall, Englewood Cliffs, New Jersey.

Kuhn T. (1970) *The Structure of Scientific Revolutions* (2nd edn). University of Chicago Press, Chicago.

Lakatos I. (1970) Falsification and the methodology of scientific research programs. In I. Lakatos & A. Musgrave (eds) *Criticism and the Growth of Knowledge*. Cambridge University Press, Cambridge.

Lancaster R. (1998) Powerful nurses protect patients. *Nursing Standard*, **13** (7), 30–31.

LoBiondo-Wood G. & Haber J. (1998) *Nursing Research*. Mosby, Missouri.

Marriner-Tomey A. (1994) *Nursing Theorists and their Work* (3rd edn). Mosby, St Louis.

Marx K. (1844) 'Paris manuscripts'. In T. Honderich (ed.) (1995) *The Oxford Companion to Philosophy*. Oxford University Press, Oxford, p. 525.

McClarey M. & Duff L. (1997) Clinical effectiveness and evidence-based practice. *Nursing Standard*, **17** (11), 31–5.

McInnes E., Cullum N., Nelson A. & Duff L. (1998) Royal College of Nursing guidelines on the management of leg ulcers. *Nursing Standard*, **13** (9), 61–3.

McKenna H. & Mason C. (1998) Nursing and the R & D agenda: Influence and contribution. *Nursing Times Research*, **3**, 108–15.

McMahon A. & Kitson A. (1997) Supporting R & D: the role of a professional organisation. *Nursing Standard* **12** (11), 36–8; and **12** (12), 35–9.

Meyer J. (1993) New paradigm research in practice: the trials and tribulations of action research. *Journal of Advanced Nursing*, **18**, 1066–72.

Miller D. (1976) *Social Justice*. Clarendon Press, Oxford.

Mitchell G. & Cody W. (1996) Nursing knowledge and human science: ontological and epistemological considerations. In J. Kenney (ed.) *Philosophical and Theoretical Perspectives for Advanced Nursing Practice*. Jones and Bartlett, London.

Moore A. (1998) Degrees of separation. *Nursing Standard*, **12** (29), 14.

Munhall P. (1982) Nursing philosophy and nursing research: In apposition or opposition? *Nursing Research*, **31**, 176–7.

Newman M. (1979) *Theory Development in Nursing*. F.A. Davis, Philadelphia.

Nichols R. (1997) Promoting action research in health care settings. *Nursing Standard*, **11** (40), 36–8.

Nightingale F. (1946) *Notes in Nursing. What It Is and What It Is Not* (orig. 1859). Lippincott, Philadelphia.

Oakley A. (1980) *Women Confined: Towards a Sociology of Childbirth*. Martin Robertson, Oxford.

Oakley A. (1984) What price professionalism? The importance of being a nurse ... obsession with professional status may prove counter-productive. *Nursing Times*, **80** (50), 24–7.

Open College (1996) *Development Studies in Nursing and Health Care. An Evolving Profession*. Multiprint Lithographics & Co., Manchester.

Orem D. (1980) *Nursing Concepts of Practice*. McGraw Hill, London.

Peplau H. (1961) *Interpersonal Relations in Nursing*. G.P. Putman & Sons, New York.

Perry A. (1993) A sociologist's view: the handmaiden's theory. In M. Jolley & G. Brykczyñska (eds) *Nursing: its Hidden Agendas*. Edward Arnold, London.

Perry A. (1997) *Nursing: A Knowledge Base for Practice* (2nd edition). Arnold, London.

Polit D. & Hungler B. (1991) *Nursing Research: Principles and Methods* (4th edn). Lippincott, Philadelphia.

Polkinghorne D. (1983) *Methodology for the Human Sciences: Systems of Inquiry*. State University of New York Press, Albany.

Popper K. (1959) *The Logic of Scientific Discovery*. Basic Books, New York.

Porter S. (1994) New nursing: the road to freedom. *Journal of Advanced Nursing*, **20**, 269–74.

Rawcliffe C. (1998) *Medieval concepts of medicine*. Lecture given at the University of East Anglia, Norwich, Wellcome Institute for the History of Medicine.

Risdale L. (1998) *Evidence-based Practice in Primary Care*. Churchill Livingstone, Edinburgh.

Roberts H. (1995) *Doing Feminist Research*. Routledge, London.

Roper N., Logan W. & Teirnay A. (1981) *Elements of Nursing*. Churchill Livingstone, London.

Roy C. (1981) *Conceptual Models for Nursing Practice* (2nd edn). Appleton Century Crofts, London.

Royal College of Nursing (1998) *What's the Evidence? Clinical Effectiveness*. Update Learning Unit 087. Royal College of Nursing Publishing, London.

Risdale L. (1995) *Evidence-based General Practice. A Critical Reader*. W.B. Saunders & Company Ltd, London.

Sackett D.L., Rosenberg W.M.C., Gray J.A.M., Haynes R.B. & Richardson W.S. (1996) Evidence-based medicine: what it is and what it isn't. *British Medical Journal*, **312**, 71–2.

Salter B. (1998) *The Politics of Change in the Health Service*. Macmillan, Basingstoke.

Salvage J. (1998) Evidence-based practice: a mixture of motives? *Nursing Times Research*, **3**, 406–18.

Schon D. (1983) *The Reflective Practitioner*. Basic Books, New York.

Schon D. (1991) *The Reflective Practitioner – How Professionals Think in Action*. Aldershot, Avebury.

Schostak J. (1998) *The PANDA (nursing practice and assessment) research project*. Personal communication.

Schratz M. & Walker R. (1995) *Research as Social Change. New Opportunities for Qualitative Research*. Routledge, London.

Sleep J. (1998) Director of the Centre for Evidence-based Practice, Wolfson Institute of Health Sciences, Thames Valley University. Presentation to the University of East Anglia School of Nursing and Midwifery. November 27.

Smith M. (1984) Research methodology: epistemologic considerations. *Image: the Journal of Nursing Scholarship*, **16** (2), 42–6.

Spender D. (1981) *Men's Studies Modified*. Pergamon Press, New York.

Starfield B. (1985) *The Effectiveness of Medical Care: Validating Clinical Wisdom*. John Hopkins University Press, London.

Sullivan P. (1998) Developing evidence-based care in mental health nursing. *Nursing Standard*, **12** (31), 35–8.

Tattam A. & Thompson M. (1993) Political influences in nursing. In M. Jolley & G. Brykczyñska (eds) *Nursing: its Hidden Agendas*. Edward Arnold, London.

Thomas L. (1998) Editorial. *Nursing Standard*, **13** (9), 1.

Thompson D. (1998) Why evidence-based nursing? *Nursing Standard*, **13** (9), 58–9.

UK Central Council for Nursing, Midwifery and Health Visiting (1992a) *Code of Professional Conduct*. UKCC Publications, London.

UK Central Council for Nursing, Midwifery and Health Visiting (1992b) *Scope of Professional Practice*. UKCC Publications, London.

UK Central Council for Nursing, Midwifery and Health Visiting (1998) *Register 25*. Autumn. UKCC Publications, London.

Visintainer M. (1996) The Nature of Knowledge and Theory in Nursing. In J. Kenney (ed.) *Philosophical and Theoretical Perspectives for Advanced Nursing Practice*. Jones & Bartlett, London.

Vredevoe D. (1984) Curology: a basic science related to nursing. *Image: the Journal of Nursing Scholarship*, **16** (3), 89–92.

Walsh M. (1997) Perceptions of barriers to implementing research. *Nursing Standard*, **11** (19), 34–7.

Walsh M. & Ford P. (1989) Rituals in nursing: 'We always do it this way', Part 1. *Nursing Times*, **85** (41), 26–32.

Webster G., Jacox A. & Baldwin B. (1981) Nursing theory and the ghost of the received view. In H. Grace & J. McCloskey (eds) *Current Issues in Nursing*. Blackwell Scientific, Boston.

Weidenbach F. (1964) *Clinical Nursing: a Helping Art*. Springer, New York.

Wesley R. (1995) *Nursing Theories and Models* (2nd edition). Springhouse Corp., Pennsylvania.

Wolfson Institute of Health Sciences Web Page (1998) http://www.wolfson.tvu.ac.uk/research/evidence/aims.html (updated 30 March 1998).

Chapter 7

Evidence-Based Practice in Social Work and Probation

Liz Trinder

Introduction

Like many other professions, social work and probation have experienced an explosion of evidence-based terminology, initiatives and publications over the last few years. These new initiatives and ideas have not, however, emerged into a methodological or research vacuum. Social work and probation have a long and frequently contested history of research into effectiveness. The recent adoption of evidence-based concepts has to be understood within the context of existing, and frequently competing research traditions within social work and probation, each of which appears to be reworking evidence-based practice within the framework of pre-existing research and practice traditions. As yet although there is considerable interest in evidence-based approaches, there is limited agreement about the definition, and even less about the potential of evidence-based practice.

The chapter begins with a summary of the nature of social work and probation, then moves onto an outline of research traditions within social work and probation, and the relationship between research and practice. The second half of the chapter tracks the emergence of evidence-based practice in this field and considers the potential and relevance of evidence-based approaches for social work and probation.

The nature of social work and probation

Social work as an enterprise is not easily summarised. Social work has always been an occupation that has suffered from something of an identity crisis, uncertain about its professional status, its function and its disciplinary base. Although something called social work occurs in many societies, its form, purpose and methods have varied considerably, moulded by the shifting influences of political/institutional contexts, intellectual traditions and social movements (Lorenz 1994). In the UK there have been ongoing debates about what social work is, with little resolution other than that social work is what social workers do (Davies 1991: 2).

The roots of social work and probation in the UK stem from a range of diverse philanthropic and voluntary activities concerning the poor in the late nineteenth century. In the first half of the twentieth century, state-funded social work activity emerged incrementally with the appearance of distinct occupational groupings with responsibility for particular client groups, including probation officers, hospital almoners and psychiatric social workers. Responsibility for children living apart from their parents remained divided between local authority public assistance departments, education departments and voluntary organisations such as Barnardos. The first social work training course was established at the London School of Economics in 1929, but the intellectual foundations of the nascent profession remained uneven (Munro 1998).

The post-war years witnessed a significant shift in the development of social work as a profession. Against the backdrop of the introduction of the Beveridge welfare state, the 1948 Children Act brought services for children together into newly formed local authority children's departments staffed by social work-trained child care officers. The early to mid-1970s represented the high watermark for the notion of a coherent social work profession in England and Wales, with the creation and rapid growth of integrated social services departments, bringing together previously separate local authority departments for children, the elderly and mental health. Work with adult offenders, however, remained the separate responsibility of local probation services under the Home Office. At the same time, the new Certificate of Qualification in Social Work (CQSW) was introduced as the first generic training for social workers and probation officers.

Although organisationally more coherent, the professional basis of social work and probation from the 1970s onwards has been contested. Attempts to produce integrated theories for social work practice (e.g. Pincus & Minahan 1973) rapidly foundered, whilst the long dominant casework approach to practice, loosely formulated within a psychoanalytic tradition, was increasingly challenged by effectiveness researchers (see following section) and the increasingly vocal radical and feminist social work movements. As Munro points out, no single theoretical framework replaced the collapse of the psychoanalytic paradigm, and there remains no clear or explicit knowledge base underpinning practice (Munro 1998: 22).

The internal critiques by radical social workers in the 1970s were rapidly matched and superseded by external critiques of social work and probation from successive Conservative governments, as well as from mounting media and public criticism of social work practice in child protection and residential child care. The corporatist self-confidence of the 1970s has been replaced by a sense of an insecure profession under siege. In the mid-1990s the training of probation officers was separated from the training of social workers, and there was no requirement for the new care managers in community care to have a social work qualification. Attempts to control the content of social work education have been highlighted in the shift towards competency-based training via the Diploma in Social Work (DipSW) (Webb 1996). Control is evident too, in the increased bureaucratisation and proceduralisation of social work, with the emphasis on assessment and risk management, plans, contracts and checklists (Howe 1992; Parton 1996).

Nonetheless, social work or social care remains a large, if extremely diverse field of activity (see Box 7.1). It is worth noting that only 40 000 of social work's one-million-strong workforce are qualified social workers. The probation workforce is much smaller.

Box 7.1: Social work and probation – key data

Social workers' work includes:

- child protection and family support
- children and adults with physical and learning disabilities
- young offenders
- mental health
- the elderly.

Probation officers work with:

- adult offenders
- families where there are disputes about children's residence and contact after divorce.

In 1996/97, public expenditure on the personal social services in England was £9.3 billion, a quarter of expenditure on the NHS (Department of Health 1998a).

In the same period 229 442 people (full-time equivalent) were employed by social services departments (DoH 1998b).

The 54 English and Welsh probation services employed 14 831 FTEs in 1997, half of which were on probation grades (probation officers and managers) (Home Office 1998b).

The total sector social care workforce is currently about one million, two-thirds of whom are in the private sector (HMSO 1998: 5.1).

The social care workforce is extremely diverse, and includes qualified social workers, managers and policy-makers, occupational therapists, social work assistants, registration and inspection staff, care managers, drivers and escorts, home helps, care staff, drugs and alcohol workers, guardians *ad litem*, nursery officers and teachers.

Approximately 80% of the workforce have no recognised qualifications or training (HMSO 1998: 5.1).

The research and practice background

The history of research in social work and probation

Research and evaluation has had a long but contested history in social work and probation. Although social workers were among the first to evaluate interventions, nevertheless the nature and role of research has continued to generate intense and often acrimonious exchanges. Debate, in both the US and UK, has frequently been polarised between experimental/empirical and non-experimental camps. These methodological debates are embedded in deeper unresolved debates about the theoretical basis and purpose of social work. The diverse roots of social work have precluded the emergence of a homogeneous disciplinary or theoretical basis for practice. Instead there is a multiplicity of theories drawing from a wide range of disciplines, with divergent focuses (Goldstein 1986) underpinned by divergent methodological traditions (see Box 7.2).

Box 7.2: Research traditions in social work and probation

Empirical Practice: emphasis on experimental designs – randomised controlled trials (RCTs), meta-analysis and single-case designs. Focus on identifying the relative effectiveness of different interventions.

Pragmatism: primarily non-experimental quantitative designs supplemented by qualitative research. Focus on identifying how systems work and their outcomes.

Empowerment/Critical: primarily qualitative designs. Focus on using research to highlight and challenge inequality.

(see Trinder 1996)

The early years to 'nothing works'

The early years of social work research, in the late nineteenth and early twentieth centuries were dominated by qualitative case studies of individual clients (Tyson 1995). The experimental tradition began in the USA in the 1930s with a major study on preventing delinquency (Powers & Witmer 1951). The formation of the Social Work Research Group in the USA in the 1950s gave a further thrust to an experimental, 'scientific' approach to social work, based on the application of findings from randomised controlled trials (Tyson 1995). Although this methodological approach was far from universally accepted, the substantive findings were highly influential as a succession of studies reported that social work and probation methods were ineffective (e.g. Mullen & Dumpson 1972; Segal 1972; Fischer 1973, 1976; Martinson 1974; Lipton *et al.* 1975; Folkard *et al.* 1976; Wood 1978). For both social work and probation the 'nothing works' conclusion drawn from these experimental studies (Martinson 1974) dealt a devastating blow to the self-esteem and rehabilitative ideals of a profession committed to helping people, and particularly to the dominant approach of psychoanalytic casework.

From 'nothing works' to 'something works'

The response to the 'nothing works' message was diverse. For the experimental or empirical practice movement it produced a renewed effort to prove that the *right* things did work, at least if rigorously measured. The movement placed enormous emphasis on encouraging practitioners to evaluate their own practice in a rigorous way, particularly through single-case designs (see Hersen & Barlow 1976; Bloom & Block 1977; Blyth & Briar 1985). At the same time, a new generation of group experimental designs began to report more positive findings about social work effectiveness, particularly those based on more structured methods of intervention, such as cognitive–behavioural therapy, rather than the loosely defined casework approach (e.g. Reid & Hanrahan 1980, 1982; Rubin 1985; Thomlinson 1984; Videka-Sherman 1988; Macdonald & Sheldon 1992).

Yet the positive findings and cohort of single case study textbooks has not amounted to Fischer's (1981) trumpeting of a 'social work revolution'. Effectiveness is now inescapably on the agenda in social work and probation, as with all other areas of social intervention, but an army of empirical practitioners has failed to materialise (Witkin 1996). In the US, the empirical practice movement remains one approach amongst many, whilst in the UK despite a considerable impact of the 'what works' movement in probation, the mainstream of social work research continues to be dominated by other traditions (Trinder 1996). Despite prolonged and impassioned pleas, UK advocates of empirical practice have, at least until recently, been effectively marginalised (see Sheldon 1983, 1986; Macdonald & Sheldon 1992; Macdonald 1994, 1996; Macdonald & Roberts 1995). Reported single case designs have been exceedingly few (for an exception see Kazi & Wilson 1996).

Effectiveness and pragmatism

In both the US, and especially the UK, the empirical practice movement has remained a minority, if organised, voice. In the UK most research, and most research on effectiveness, fits within a broad pragmatist approach. For pragmatists, research design is based on technical rather than epistemological or ontological grounds. There is a strong preference for non-experimental quantitative designs using non-randomised samples, possibly supplemented by qualitative methods in a secondary or illustrative role. Though the pragmatists have not been formally united by a manifesto in the same way as the empirical practice movement has, there is a significant degree of *de facto* commonality, including broadly shared views on practice, research design, methods and epistemology. Grand science and grand experimental designs are cut down to size within a realist epistemological framework. For Roger Fuller this means 'the suspension of not-to-be-resolved philosophical conundra in the interests of getting on with the job' (Fuller 1996: 59), leading to a trade-off between what is desirable and what is feasible, and abandoning the search for irrefutable scientific proof (Fuller 1996: 59). The majority of the major research studies in the UK would probably fit within this non-experimental tradition, including research funded by the Department of Health in child care and community care (e.g. Cheetham *et al.* 1992; Fuller & Petch 1995; Dartington Social Research Unit 1995; Social Work Research Centre 1998).

Empowerment and effectiveness

A third empowerment-orientated tradition in social work research drawing on interpretivist or critical theory has been a continuing if less influential approach. In contrast to empirical practice and pragmatist research, empowerment or participative/critical research has an explicitly political focus. The early qualitative studies in social work (e.g. Mayer & Timms 1970; Sainsbury 1975) drew on an interpretative tradition in seeking (for what seemed the first time) the subjective meanings clients gave to events and experiences. Over the last few years this relativist position has shifted towards a more radical and critical stance using the research process and research findings to challenge structural inequalities. For participative/critical researchers the research act, like social work practice, is about power and empowerment. Research is not posited as a neutral fact-finding activity. Instead research, researchers and research participants are located within a world where power is unequally distributed between genders, classes, ethnic groups, professionals and clients. Research can therefore be used to ignore, reinforce or, preferably for participative/critical researchers, to identify and challenge inequalities. To achieve the latter there is a (varying) emphasis on the involvement of research participants in typically small-scale qualitative studies, as well as using research findings as a means to empower disadvantaged groups (e.g. Hart & Bond 1995; Everitt & Hardiker 1996). This research approach is explicitly linked to the radical, feminist and anti-oppressive approaches to social work (Trinder 1996).

Within this tradition the notion of effectiveness is viewed with some suspicion. Harrison & Humphries (1997), for example, express concern about the linkages between new managerialism and effectiveness, and the threat this poses to a critical knowledge base within social work. Their definition of research-mindedness includes 'a faculty for critical reflection informed by knowledge and research which is inextricably allied to practice which counters unfair discrimination, racism, poverty, disadvantage and injustice and core social work values' (Harrison & Humphries 1997: 8).

Practitioners and the use of research

Although social work research is acknowledged to have had a significant impact on policy, the relationship between research and practice appears to be much more limited (Independent Review Group 1994; Munro 1998). Although some studies have found that a high proportion of social workers reported using research (e.g. Sinclair & Jacobs 1995), the majority of studies highlight the greater influence of intuition, values and practice wisdom (Parsloe & Stevenson 1978; Corby 1982; Social Services Inspectorate 1993). Munro (1998) identifies a supermarket approach to social work theory where a whole range of competing perspectives are presented to students with no empirical indication of their relative effectiveness. Not surprisingly, students and social workers do not use either theory or research systematically or fluently (Secker 1993; Munro 1998). Munro argues that where good data is available social workers persist in ignoring it as part of what she terms an anti-scientific ethos in social work (Munro 1998: 25–6). A study by Macdonald (1994) similarly found that probation officers assessed and intervened on the basis of their own favoured theory or perspective, ignoring alternative approaches. Humphrey and Pease's (1992) study of probation officers found that effectiveness was not discussed, or was viewed in terms of inputs (producing a report which resulted in the court making a probation order) rather than outputs (the results of the probation order).

There are a number of reasons for the limited usage of research in social work. Although research awareness remains part of the CCETSW (Central Council for Education and Training in Social Work) qualifying requirements for the DipSW (Diploma in Social Work) and part of the BASW (British Association of Social Workers) Code of Ethics, limited time is available on training courses for research training (CCETSW/PSSC 1980; Harrison & Humphries 1997).

Even if research training were more prevalent, there is a limited amount of research available. Personal social services research has always been the poor relation of health services research, with proportionately less funding (CCETSW/PSSC 1980; Independent Review Group 1994). Funding is currently split between the Department of Health, universities, charities and social services departments. There is no regional research and development structure equivalent to that in health research. The consequence is an overall shortage of research, with Glisson & Fischer (1987) calculating that less than 45% of articles in major social work journals were based on empirical research findings. There are also concerns over the quality of research. Gibbons & Tunstill (1993) noted that peer review was not always effective in personal social services research, and argued for improved mechanisms to ensure reliability and validity. Macdonald and Sheldon (1992), in their review of effectiveness, found only 95 studies which met their methodological criteria, which though strict for social work, were relaxed compared to those of the Cochrane Collaboration.

The limited amount of good quality research is compounded by problems with dissemination. Despite some acclaimed collations of research in particular areas (e.g. DHSS 1985; Department of Health 1991), dissemination has been uncoordinated (Gibbons & Tunstill 1993) and under-resourced (Independent Review Group 1994). Consequently access to research findings is restricted.

The emergence and development of evidence-based practice

The rapid development of evidence-based practice in the health field has generated a fair degree of interest in the associated areas of social work and probation. A powerful advocate for this transmigration was the then secretary of state for health, Stephen Dorrell:

> 'The commitment to evidence-based medicine increasingly pervades modern medical practice. This kind of commitment should be extended to the social services world'.
>
> (Dorrell 1996)

The response to such an appeal has been fragmented and has to be understood in the context of pre-existing research traditions within social work and probation. Two fairly distinctive approaches are beginning to emerge, one associated with the empirical practice lobby and one associated with a more mainstream pragmatist group of researchers. Both have adopted the language of evidence-based practice, and some of its concepts, and melded them into their existing approaches.

Experimental versions of evidence-based practice

The empirical practice movement within social work and the associated what-works movement in criminology/probation share many of the aims, methods and enthusiasms of the evidence-based practice movement in health, specifically the emphasis on basing interventions on research evidence derived from randomised controlled trials (RCTs) and meta-analysis. Both indigenous movements have explicitly associated themselves with the evidence-based practice originating in the health field.

The two most prominent advocates of empirical practice in the UK, Geraldine Macdonald and Brian Sheldon, have explicitly adopted the evidence-based tag. Macdonald, a former Cochrane Fellow, has written extensively, if at times despairingly, of the need for RCTs and evidence-based social work (Macdonald 1997a,b). Sheldon now heads a centre for evidence-based social services, established in April 1997, funded jointly by the Department of Health and 19 social services departments in the south-west of England on £2.5 million over three years. The decision to include 'evidence-based' in the centre's title was deliberately prompted by Sheldon as a means to emulate and link into developments in medicine and health care (personal communication). The centre has three main functions:

(1)   To carry out or commission studies in areas where there are significant gaps in knowledge.
(2)   To disseminate research on the origins and development of social problems and on the effectiveness of different approaches to them.
(3)   To provide training in interpreting and using research findings to inform practice.

In probation the development of evidence-based approaches has progressed further. Over the last decade, work with offenders has become far more focused on the clear goal of confronting offending behaviour and reducing recidivism, rather than a more general social work approach placing greater emphasis on a client's social situation. Supporting, and partly driving this focus, has been the emergence of a comprehensive body of research from administrative criminology with clear, coherent research-based messages about what works in reducing offending and recidivism (see Underdown 1988 for a summary). Policy-makers and probation managers have rapidly adopted the emphasis on what works. The Home Office Inspectorate of Probation 'What Works' project (subsequently the Effective Practice Initiative) draws heavily on largely North American RCT and meta-analysis findings on interventions to reduce offending. A national implementation strategy for the project is now under way, incorporating staff training and development and the accreditation of programmes, and national standards for practice are being drafted (Probation Circular 35/98 June). A recent practice guide from the project is significantly entitled *Evidence-Based Practice: A Guide to Effective Practice*, covering all aspects of what works from practice to management (Home Office 1988a).

Pragmatist versions of evidence-based practice

The empirical practice and what-works camps are not the only ones who are promoting evidence-based social work. The pragmatists, in classically pragmatic fashion, have also adopted the language of evidence-based practice, though with little of the associated technical and methodological apparatus. This neat move has not gone unnoticed by Geraldine Macdonald who has expressed concern about the adoption of a much looser definition of evidence, and denial of a hierarchy of evidence by key figures, including the social services section of the Department of Health (Macdonald 1997a,b).

One of the key figures in the pragmatist camp is Michael Little from Dartington, who has argued for a more global understanding of evidence-based social work based on a range of research, including RCTs on effectiveness, but also his own framework, *Matching Needs and Services*, for profiling service needs (Little 1998: 53). Thus:

> 'Dartington has tried to outline the beginning of a common conceptual framework in what it calls evidence-based social work. This seeks to link concepts of need, threshold, service and outcome in the study, management and clinical practice of children's services.'
>
> (Little 1998: 53)

The joint Dartington–Sheffield University Research in Practice project runs with the slogan 'Towards evidence-based work with children and families', and has the stated aim of promoting 'evidence-based practice and policy in child welfare services'. The project is an Association of Directors of Social Services initiative, with a membership of fee-paying social services departments and voluntary organisations. Its primary aims are to disseminate research findings to managers and practitioners and to enhance critical appraisal skills. The project runs seminars and workshops and also has a computerised directory of research findings. The directory, like the dissemination seminars, does not distinguish between types of evidence. The consortium, Making Research Count, based at five universities (East Anglia, Leicester, Luton, Royal Holloway, York) is also focusing on research dissemination, again within a broadly pragmatist rather than empirical practice framework.

Divergent and convergent approaches

There are, therefore, two camps in social work and probation currently claiming to be evidence-based. For the pragmatists, evidence-based means essentially research-based practice, drawing on a range of different types of research, including RCTs where available. There is no attempt to create a hierarchy of evidence of effectiveness with RCTs located at the top. In contrast, the empirical practice/what-works camp draws almost exclusively on an experimental tradition, thus aligning it much more closely to the classic medicine and Cochrane definition of evidence-based practice.

In practice, however, significant differences exist between the empirical practice/what-works approaches and that of evidence-based practice in health care (see Chapters 3, 4 and 5). In terms of social work the lack of available trial data requires an approach more akin to that of the pragmatists. Brian Sheldon, for example, whilst admiring the Cochrane approach, acknowledged in an interview with the author that the typical Cochrane inclusion criteria would result in the elimination of almost all social work research. He therefore reluctantly favours a pragmatic pyramid-of-certainty approach, with successive levels of confidence attributed to different research designs, with RCTs at the top, followed by quasi-experiments, pre post-test and so on. The inability to rely simply on RCT evidence does not just extend to existing research. None of the four major research projects for which Sheldon's Centre for Evidence-Based Social Services was seeking tenders, included an RCT.

In probation the what-works/effective practice initiative approach also diverges from classic evidence-based practice approaches in health. Here more trial data is available on interventions with adult offenders. However, rather than an approach which begins with the individual case and formulation of an answerable question and then proceeds to a search for relevant research evidence, in probation the thrust is towards providing a single approach, or magic solution, to all problems. The Home Office Inspectorate of Probation Effective Practice initiative, particularly the recently issued *Evidence-Based Practice: a Guide to Effective Practice* (HMSO 1998), presents such a prescriptive approach to practice based on social learning theories, especially cognitive–behavioural approaches and social skills training. The implication is that in all situations, with all clients, a similar approach should be adopted. Although the research evidence suggests that social learning approaches tend to be more effective in reducing recidivism (Ross & Fabiano 1985; Andrews *et al.* 1990; Palmer 1995), the evidence is by no means unequivocal or conclusive (e.g. Whitehead & Lab 1989; Pannizon *et al.* 1991), and certainly does not support a universal generic approach to practice.

Can evidence-based practice work in social work and probation?

Evidence-based approaches have then arrived in social work and probation. As yet their influence is fairly marginal, and most practitioners, particularly in social work, will be unaware of their presence. The question then arises as to how useful and relevant is evidence-based practice? We have already seen how evidence-based practice, as conceived in medicine, has altered its character in the transfer to both empirical practice and pragmatist approaches to social work and probation. Is this a dangerous dilution of principle, as Macdonald (1997b) fears, weakening the potential of evidence-based practice before it even starts? Or is there something distinctive about the nature of social work and probation, which necessitates some deviation from the classic formulation of evidence-based practice? Will evidence-based practice result in a potentially reductionist approach to practice, or enhance the effectiveness of practice?

Certainly there are compelling reasons for the greater use of evidence of effectiveness. Social workers and probation officers work with some of the most vulnerable as well as the more dangerous members of society, and have an ethical duty to offer the most effective help. The well-documented failures in child protection and residential care, and inconsistency in practice have led to proposals for a new General Social Care Council for social work and a range of measures to raise standards in the latest White Paper, *Modernising Social Services* (HMSO 1998). Researchers from pragmatist and empirical camps are agreed on the need to produce evidence to both protect and enhance social work and probation (e.g. Cheetham *et al.* 1992; Macdonald 1996; Munro 1998). But would a fully evidence-based practice make a difference? Is evidence-based social work and probation possible, and if it is, is it desirable?

It is here that we are forced to confront the real world of practice. My argument is that social work and probation are not the same as medicine, where the physiological effect of an intervention dose is relatively predictable from person to person and where, to a far greater extent, extraneous factors can be excluded. In crude terms, the medical implication is in situation A, do B to achieve result C. In contrast, encounters between social workers and their clients involve human relationships rather than pharmacological or physical interventions. Social work and probation clients come with their own histories and understandings, and are embedded in continuing social relationships, with family, friends and colleagues, outside of the context of the intervention. They are not passive recipients of an intervention, but are actively engaging or disengaging. Furthermore, the issue or problem is not detached or detachable, but typically multifactorial and impacting on and engaging with other aspects of the person's life. Despite the current emphasis in probation on working on the 'distorted thinking patterns' of offenders, the influence of other factors – housing, employment, and poverty – remains vitally important (Raynor *et al.* 1994). Even if there were a single isolated issue to work on, the process of engagement will, of necessity, require a complex sequence of human relationships. In summary, social work encounters are not straightforward or linear relationships, but multiple, multilayered, relational and complex, and located in a social and political context. Within this framework of the inherently messy and complex nature of social work and probation relationships, classic formulations of evidence are impoverished and potentially constraining.

I want to pursue these arguments further, not arguing against evidence, but for the kind of evidence that does justice to individual cases. I will look at three main issues: the current lack of evidence; the epistemological and ontological assumptions of evidence-based/empirical practice approaches; and the limited potential of RCTs to focus on the vital questions of what it is which makes an intervention work or not work. My argument is not against evidence, but for a type of evidence-based practice that will generate ideas about effectiveness, which are useful to practitioners, based on good quality evidence implemented by highly reflective and reflexive practitioners.

Lack of evidence

In most areas of social work practice, though to a lesser extent in probation, there is very little trial data available. The recent series of *What Works* summaries produced by Barnardos was intended to focus on RCT evidence. Yet in most areas, the data simply are not available (e.g. Sellick & Thoburn 1997; Stein 1997). Even in the US, where empirical social work research is at its most advanced, the outcomes of experimental and quasi-experimental studies have yielded comparatively little fruit. A recent summary of US research into child welfare outcomes by a leading authority (Maluccio 1998) contains two key messages. First, that across a whole range of studies the findings are inconclusive. Second, that studies are bedevilled by methodological problems of inadequate control, underspecified experimental (i.e. nature of the intervention) and outcome variables. The similarly well-developed literature on crime prevention has produced equally ambiguous messages (Pawson 1997).

Technical issues

It would be tempting to blame social work researchers and funders, educators and practitioners for the lack of evidence and the lack of use of what hard evidence is available. On this basis a rapid and thorough research programme, coupled with an intensive training programme, might make evidence-based practice possible in the near future. Whilst there may be some truth in that, in other ways, the world in which practitioners operate simply makes straightforward questions and answers extremely difficult to find.

There are a number of technical issues that make RCTs more difficult to operationalise within social work and probation than medicine. Ethical and practical problems make randomised allocation of subjects a comparatively rare event (Maluccio 1998). Second, disentangling causes or excluding confounding variables is also more challenging given that research participants are not hermetically sealed from influences other than the intervention, many or most of which the practitioners or researchers will remain unaware. It can, therefore, be difficult to identify what causes change. The third, technical issue to raise is the generally contested nature of outcome indicators. It is seldom possible to find an agreed outcome measure that can capture all dimensions of change. Instead, fairly crude approximations are often used: in crime it is often reconviction rates, which are notoriously inaccurate (Mair *et al.* 1997); in studies of child placement (adoption and fostering), it is placement breakdown rates.

There is, of course, a strong argument that these technical difficulties strengthen rather than weaken the case for RCTs, that the power and neutrality of a well-designed RCT is specifically designed to cope with this 'noise' or variations in the internal and external worlds of clients. This argument has considerable force, but I want to argue that the scope for RCTs within social work and probation will remain limited for technical reasons. There are also other serious questions, firstly about the neutrality of RCTs as a research technology, and secondly about the ability of RCTs and meta-analyses to provide useful information on the crucial question of which interventions work for which people and why.

Beyond the microscope: epistemological issues

My argument so far has been that a particular version of science is a blunt or brutal instrument for dealing with the complexity of human behaviour, emotions and relationships. Extending this further it is possible that the apparent cleanliness and transparency of science may go beyond failing to do justice to complexity, and may even simplify and distort the picture that is seen, with significant consequences for practice.

On this point, Witkin (1994) disputes the claim of theory and practice neutrality of the American empirical practice movement (e.g. Bloom *et al.* 1995). Instead he argues that the toolkit of RCTs, meta-analyses and single case designs, is located within an unacknowledged value system or meta-theory, which generates or shapes the reality it seeks to discover and change. Thus attempts to exclude politics, bias and noise through the technology of the RCT and meta-analysis are themselves part of a meta-theory, which renders the world as orderly, rational, clean, certain and safe. The mechanisms of empirical practice conceptualise individuals as self-contained units acted on by external forces, rather than individuals as products of relational forces:

> 'The structural constraints imposed by empirical metatheory favor certain forms of understanding over others. Empirical practice supports explanations of social life that are deterministic, easily measurable, and adaptable to single-system designs. It tends to suppress alternative ways of understanding that cannot accommodate these constraints – for example, narrative accounts. These differ-

ences have implications for how we think about human beings and their problems and how people think about themselves'.

(Witkin 1996: 73)

As Howe (1997) points out, such a conception of the rational and autonomous rather than the social and relational self is closely embedded in the
contemporary political context of welfare, and the contemporary dominance of libertarian individualism, with its focus on autonomy, self-
determination and individual rights and responsibilities. Hence practice
tends to be rational, problem-focused, with 'behavioural objectives, measured outcomes, agreements and legal-like contracts to organise and
manage social relationships' in contrast to conceptualising individuals as
emotional, relational, confused and conflicted (Howe 1997: 166).

As we have seen above, social work lacks a single body of knowledge or
theory. This is not a reflection on the quality of social work theorists or
researchers but a reflection of the complexity of the situations with which
social workers deal. In terms of assessment, should the focus be, as Munro
(1988) asks, on structural factors (poverty, housing and so on); or on
behavioural patterns, attachments or childhood experiences; or a combination of each? In terms of intervention, Goldstein questions:

> 'Should the focus be on the client's ego strengths, social role, psychosocial pat-
> terns, personality traits, or status in his or her system? Or, should the focus be on
> the family's interactions, communication patterns, selected external re-enforce-
> ments, or what?'

(Goldstein 1986: 354)

In complex situations there are real difficulties in identifying single
answerable questions or providing straightforward questions. The questions asked and answers provided will depend to a great extent on what
vantage point or theoretical perspective is taken. Inevitably therefore some
potentially significant questions and answers will be excluded, the risk of
which may be greater where there is little or no evidence.

Complexity is also smoothed out in the sense that the empirical practice
movement and its associated methodological technology also seek to
achieve a single truth, a single objective verdict on particular interventions.
The more the evidence-based process is refined, the greater the sense, or
claim that it is safer, more reliable, and closer to the truth. Yet we know that
the social world is full of multiple perspectives. Smith and Cantley's (1985)
classic study of a psychogeriatric day hospital demonstrated how divergent views could be on the definition of what a successful outcome would
be between different professional groups and between professionals and
carers.

Despite a welcome emphasis within the Cochrane Collaboration's work
on consumer participation, it is clear that the issues important to con-

sumers may well differ from those important to professionals and researchers. Oliver (1997: 276), for example, identifies a mismatch between the broader definition of health held by lay people and the narrow definition adopted by researchers, leading them to adopt a narrower range of health indicators. The example is important in that it demonstrates that the research process, even when working to the strictest standards of the Cochrane Collaboration, involves making choices and interpretations. In the world of social work and probation, where the principal tool available to the practitioner is understanding and relationship-building, the reduction of a client to a set of measurable variables, and the potentially limited attention to the client's own perspectives could lead to impoverished or myopic practice.

Disaggregating the aggregate

The criticisms so far levelled at empirical practice and RCTs have been both pragmatic: that RCTs are too technically difficult in the messy world of human relationships; and epistemological, that RCTs and meta-analysis are not neutral tools and contain implicit and unacknowledged worldviews. Supporters of empirical or evidence-based practice could simply dispute both arguments, and counter that even if the criticisms had some validity that RCTs are the closest we can achieve to accuracy.

The final issue I want to raise therefore is about the limited ability of RCTs, and hence meta-analysis, to provide help to practitioners in identifying what interventions might work with which people in which conditions. As yet there are few high-quality RCTs of direct relevance to social work, and even fewer systematic reviews. Those that are available, however, provide limited guidance on which interventions will work in which conditions with which people, or *why* these interventions work. Barlow's (1998) systematic review of training programmes for parents of children with behaviour problems, for example, suggests that behavioural and group, rather than individual types of approaches tend to work best. But Barlow also concludes that, as yet, we have much less understanding of the reasons for change, or how to match interventions to individuals.

This limited purchase on matching intervention and client, or why interventions work (that is, what are the mechanisms that make a difference, and with whom), is clearly of critical importance if research is to be useful for practitioners working with individual clients. It is a problem, however, which is inherent in experimental designs. We noted above how ambiguous experimental studies have been. Pawson (1997), citing Nuttall (1992), notes the classic aggregate net-effect problem with experimental designs, whereby the positive effects for some are cancelled out by the negative effects for others in the production of a mean score. Although RCTs can identify which interventions are broadly more effective than others, or no intervention, they give limited purchase on the impact on individuals or explanations for change, or lack of change.

Yet it becomes very easy for practitioners, and managers especially it would seem, to become transfixed by the term evidence and the promise of a clear and single answer to difficult questions. In probation, the relatively greater effectiveness reported with approaches based on social learning theories has led to an almost exclusive emphasis on these approaches, and a focus on challenging distorted thinking patterns (e.g. Home Office 1998a). However, no researcher presumably would argue that social learning approaches work best in all cases.

In response to these criticisms, Ray Pawson (1997) has argued persuasively for 'scientific realist evaluation' in place of experimental designs in crime reduction programmes. His argument is that involvement in a social programme does not involve a singular treatment or dose, but rather a complex series of interactions where:

> 'Potential subjects will consider a programme (or not), volunteer for it (or not), become interested (or not), cooperate closely (or not), stay the course (or not), learn lessons (or not), retain the lessons (or not). Programmes are thus learning processes and, as with any learning process, certain groups and individuals are much more likely to have the appropriate characteristics which will allow them to stay the course'.
>
> (Pawson 1997: 155)

Scientific realist evaluation then focuses on outcomes, but explains them by identifying the mechanisms which produce them within particular shifting and contingent contexts (Pawson 1997: 157). The worked example that Pawson provides is based on attempts to reduce recidivism through an education in prison programme. The evaluation was based on the assumption that the programme would not work in an undifferentiated way and that change would be associated with a complex interrelationship of factors. Phase 1 of the evaluation was based on qualitative interviews with practitioners to identity folk hypotheses about change, that is ideas about contexts and mechanisms. Examples of these hypotheses were: the protection hypothesis – that younger, one-off violent offenders invest in the programme to get off the wing; and the self-esteem hypothesis – those with least prior educational success would benefit most. These hypotheses were then broken down into approximately 50 variables, including age of entry into the programme, previous education, and grade progress on the course. In Phase 2, outcomes based on the 50 variables were measured and compared, not with a control group, but with a predictor scale based on risk categories of re-offence (including criminal histories, demographic factors and social background). In this process actual performance could be compared with expected performance, not just in aggregate terms but focusing on the complex interrelationship of variables accounting for the outcomes of particular individuals whilst still taking account of risk levels when measuring success.

Examples of methodologies like this go beyond outcome and descriptive process evaluations and seek answers to question of what is it about the programme that works for whom? They will not be the only ones which may provide solid and relevant evidence for practitioners.

The future for evidence-based social work

This discussion has so far concentrated on some of the potential limitations or pitfalls with evidence-based practice. We now turn to the wider question of its likely future. What are its prospects? Does it have a future? Will practice become evidence-based?

It is here that probation and social work are likely to part company further. The signs at the moment are that there is likely to be a much stronger central push for evidence-based practice in probation rather than in social work. The probation field of activity is far more con-centrated on a single group of people than the disaggregated target group found in social work. The sole exception to the focus on adult offenders, the work of the family court welfare officers, historically located almost by accident within probation, is to be hived off to a sepa-rate agency within the next few years.

In social work, the position is somewhat different. There is nothing like the same degree of coherence in the focus of the work, the research or evidence base or the policy/managerial agenda. As we noted at the beginning of this chapter, social work covers a very diverse field of activity. The research base is similarly fragmented. Although in some areas of social work there is a fairly extensive body of research, in many areas there is very little. Unlike probation, where there is a clear body of research into what works, crudely summed up as cognitive–behavioural therapy, the social work research literature has not produced, and would appear unlikely to produce, a similarly coherent approach to practice. At the same time, it has to be recognised that the majority of the social care workforce has no formal qualifications and training, and there is nothing like the same degree of commitment from above to pushing evidence-based practice.

At present, efforts to push evidence-based social work are relatively dispersed. The research dissemination initiatives that are being undertaken and have Department of Health/Association of Directors of Social Services support are comparatively small, and are not working within a single definition of what constitutes evidence-based practice or even evidence. There is nothing like the coherence and drive of probation's 'what works'/ effective-practice initiative nor, in the health field, the NHS Centre for Reviews and Dissemination.

The lack of a clear Department of Health thrust towards, or prioritisation of, evidence-based social work is evident in the White Paper on *Modernising Social Services* (HMSO 1988). The 'third way' to improve the quality and outcomes of social care are clearly set within the framework of standard setting, regulation and inspection rather than evidence-based practice. The White Paper notes the presence of good practice but its overall message is that a lack of clarity about objectives and standards has resulted in much poor practice, inconsistency and inefficiency. The solution focuses primarily on procedural or process issues – setting out standards for practice, objective-setting, audit and inspection. One major innovation, again within a procedural framework, is the introduction of the new General Social Care Council to begin the process of creating a register of social care staff and to set enforceable standards of conduct and practice. The two key objectives of the GSCC are:

- 'to strengthen public protection by relevant and appropriate regulation of personnel which has the interests of service users and the public at its heart
- to ensure through a coherent, well-developed and regulated training system that more staff are equipped to provide social care which allows and assists individuals to live their own lives, and offers practical help, based on research and other evidence of what works, and free of unnecessary ideological influences'.

(HMSO 1988: para 5.15)

A new training organisation for personal social services will also be established to identify training needs and to see that they are met (HMSO 1988: para 5.34).

These new initiatives are to be welcomed but they also indicate just how much work needs to be done. Social care staff are to be registered for the first time, but acknowledging the heterogeneity of the largely unqualified workforce, the registration process will be an incremental one beginning with the 40 000 qualified social workers (HMSO 1988: paras 5.19–24). The registration of the remainder of the one-million-strong workforce will follow the identification of training needs, the creation and achievement of appropriate qualifications.

The White Paper notes:

'As in other professions, it is important that professionally qualified social workers base their practice on the best evidence of what works for clients and are responsive to new ideas from research. Their early education and training will play a significant part in encouraging a flexible, intelligent approach to practice in later years and assist social workers in taking personal responsibility for their continuing professional education and development'.

(HMSO 1988: para 5.32)

The realisation of the goal of qualified, research-literate evidence-based practitioners must, however, be some time away. In overall terms the emphasis on research and evidence in the White Paper is marginal. There are no plans to establish a research infrastructure in social work on a par with other aspects of the NHS or within probation. The future of social work is located much more firmly within a managerial–procedural discourse than a scientific evidential one.

Conclusion

The broad fields of social care and probation have a curious relationship with evidence-based practice. On the one hand, the probation service appears to have completely embraced the 'what works' movement, a movement which has developed separately from, but with many parallels with the evidence-based practice movement in health. On the other hand, the response from social work researchers has been to absorb the language of evidence-based practice into their lexicon. For the small band of empirical practitioners this has been a relatively straightforward translation, as many of the premises and techniques of evidence-based practice match quite closely the long-standing concerns of the empirical practitioners. For the pragmatists, the adoption of the language of evidence-based practice appears to be a more tactical move, incorporating the rhetorical power of the word evidence while continuing to draw upon a much wider definition of what constitutes evidence. Nonetheless, as we have seen above, whilst social care researchers are adopting the language of evidence the prospect of a fully evidence-based social work, of either a more traditional or pragmatist variety, does appear a long way off. The indications are for social work that managerial rather than scientific discourse is currently driving the government agenda.

The question then arises as to which is the better way forward, the 'what works' route of probation or the managerial emphasis in social care? There appear to be dangers in both routes. In the former there is a danger of an overly rigid practice which fails to do justice to the complexity of individual cases, where practitioners will, having been supplied with an answer, stop asking questions. On the other hand, a managerial or procedural approach to practice may fail to take advantage of what can be known about effectiveness.

The challenge for both social work/care and probation is to move beyond polarised debates about methodology. Clearly a range of types of evidence is required, including meta-analysis, RCTs and single-case designs, as well as scientific realist evaluations, research on social work processes and qualitative research. More effective dissemination is also required. Practitioners also need to be schooled in appraising research, not just in terms of assessing methodological rigour, but crucially also in thinking through how research can be utilised flexibly and reflexively in individual cases.

Nonetheless, even with a rapid increase in the quantity and quality of research in social care and probation, evidence will always remain a small part of the answer. In the field of social care and probation it is seldom possible to translate a piece of research directly to the circumstances of a particular case. There will always remain, possibly even more so than in medicine, a crucial role for the practitioner's experience and judgement. There are other considerations as well: the views and wishes of service users are rightly now also getting the recognition they deserve; alongside that, practitioners also need to consider other issues, crucially resource issues, but also moral and ethical ones (Munro 1998; Little 1998: 53).

The benefit of evidence-based practice for social care is that it has brought a welcome emphasis on research and effectiveness. The potential danger is that the rhetorical force of the word evidence, particularly evidence defined narrowly as that based on RCTs, can offer seductively simplistic messages for practitioners and managers.

References

Andrews D., Zinger I., Hoge R., Bonta J., Gendreau P. & Cullen F. (1990) Does correctional treatment work? A clinically relevant and psychologically informed meta-analysis. *Criminology*, **28**, 417–29.

Barlow J. (1998) *Systematic Review of the Effectiveness of Parent-Training Programmes in Improving Behaviour Problems in Children Aged 3–10 Years*. University of Oxford, Health Services Research Unit, Oxford.

Bloom M. & Block S. (1977) Evaluating one's own effectiveness and efficiency. *Social Work*, **22**, 130–36.

Bloom M., Fischer J. & Orme J. (1995) *Evaluating Practice: Guidelines for the Accountable Professional* (2nd edition). Allyn & Bacon, Needham Heights.

Blythe B. & Briar S. (1985) Developing empirically based models of practice. *Social Work*, **30**, 483–8.

Blythe B., Tripodi T. & Briar S. (1994) *Direct Practice Research in Human Service Agencies*. Columbia University Press, New York.

CCETSW/PSSC (1980) *Research and practice. Report of a Working Party on a Research Strategy for the Personal Social Services*. CCETSW/PSSC, London.

Cheetham J., Fuller R., Mclvor G. & Petch A. (1992) *Evaluating Social Work Effectiveness*. Open University Press, Buckingham.

Corby B. (1982) Theory and practice in long-term social work. *British Journal of Social Work*, **12**, 619–38.

Dartington Social Research Unit (1995) *Child Protection: Messages from Research*. HMSO, London.

Department of Health (1991) *Patterns and Outcomes in Child Placement*. HMSO, London.

Department of Health (1998a) Statistical Bulletin. *Personal Social Services: Current and Capital Expenditure in England: 1996–97.* DoH, London.

Department of Health (1998b) Statistical Bulletin. *Personal Social Services: Staff of Social Services Departments at 30 September 1997.* DoH, London.

DHSS (1981) *Social Work: A Research Review,* HMSO Research Report No.8. HMSO, London.

DHSS (1985) *Social Work Decisions in Child Care: Recent Research Findings and their Implications.* HMSO, London.

Dorrell S. (1996) *The Guardian,* 19 June.

Everitt A. & Hardiker P. (1996) *Evaluating for Good Practice.* Macmillan, Basingstoke.

Fischer J. (1973) Is casework effective? *Social Work,* **18**, 5–20.

Fischer J. (1976) *The Effectiveness of Social Casework.* Charles C. Thomas, Springfield, Illinois.

Fischer J. (1981) The social work revolution. *Social Work,* **26**, 199–207.

Fischer J. & Corcoran K. (1994) *Measures for Clinical Practice: a Sourcebook* (2nd edition, Vols 1 & 2). Free Press, New York.

Folkard M.S., Smith D.E. & Smith D.D. (1976) *IMPACT. The Results of the Experiment.* Home Office Research Study Number 36. HMSO, London.

Fuller R. (1996) Evaluating social work effectiveness: a pragmatic approach. In P. Alderson, S. Brill, I. Chalmers, R. Fuller & P. Hinkley-Smith (eds) *What Works? Effective Social Interventions in Child Welfare.* Barnardos, Ilford.

Fuller R. & Petch A. (1995) *Practitioner Research: The Reflexive Social Worker.* Open University Press, Buckingham.

Gibbons J. & Tunstill J. (1993) *Review of Good Dissemination Initiatives. Report to the Department of Health.* Social Work Development Unit, University of East Anglia, Norwich.

Glisson C. & Fischer J. (1987) Statistical training for social workers. *Journal of Social Work Education,* **23**, 50–58.

Goldstein H. (1986) Towards the integration of theory and practice: a humanistic approach. *Social Work,* **31**, 352–7.

Hanvey C. & Philpot T. (1996) Survival of the fittest. *Community Care,* 30 October.

Harrison C. & Humphries C. (1997) *Putting the Praxis Back into Practice: Outcomes of a survey of research-mindedness in CCETSW awards on behalf of London and South East England Region.* CCETSW, London.

Hart E. & Bond M. (1995) *Action Research for Health and Social Care: A Guide to Practice.* Open University Press, Buckingham.

Hersen M. & Barlow D.H. (1976) *Single Case Experimental Designs: Strategies for Studying Behaviour Change.* Pergamon Press, New York.

Home Office (1998a) *Evidence-Based Practice: A Guide to Effective Practice.* Home Office, London.

Home Office (1998b) *Summary Probation Statistics: England and Wales 1997.* Home Office Research and Statistics Directorate, London.

Howe D. (1992) Child abuse and the bureaucratisation of social work. *Sociological Review,* **40**, 491–508.

Howe D. (1997) Psychosocial and relationship-based theories for child and family social work: political philosophy, psychology and welfare practice. *Child and Family Social Work,* **2**, 161–70.

Humphrey C. & Pease K. (1992) Effectiveness measurement in probation: a view from the troops. *The Howard Journal*, **31**, 31–52.

Independent Review Group (1994) *A Wider Strategy for Research and Development Relating to Personal Social Services*. HMSO, London.

Kazi M. & Wilson J. (1996) Applying single-case evaluation in social work. *British Journal of Social Work*, **26**, 699–717.

Lipton D., Martinson R. & Wilkes J. (1975) *The Effectiveness of Correctional Treatment*. Praeger, New York.

Little M. (1998) Whispers in the library. *Child and Family Social Work*, **3**, 49–56.

Lorenz W. (1994) *Social Work in a Changing Europe*. Routledge, London.

Macdonald G. (1994) Developing empirically based practice in probation. *British Journal of Social Work*, **22**, 615–43.

Macdonald G. (1996) Ice therapy: why we need randomised controlled trials. In P. Alderson, S. Brill, I. Chalmers *et al.* (eds) *What Works? Effective Social Interventions in Child Welfare*. Barnardos, Barkingside.

Macdonald G. (1997a) Social work: beyond control? In A. Maynard & I. Chalmers (eds) *Non-Random Reflections on Health Services Research*. BMJ Publishing Group, London.

Macdonald G. (1997b) Social work research: the state we're in. *Journal of Inter-professional Care*, **11**, 57–65.

Macdonald G. & Roberts H. (1995) *What Works in the Early Years?* Barnardos, Ilford.

Macdonald G. & Sheldon B. (1992) Contemporary studies of the effectiveness of social work. *British Journal of Social Work*, **22**, 615–43.

Mair G., Lloyd C. & Hough M. (1997) The limitations of reconviction rates. In G. Mair (ed.) *Evaluating the Effectiveness of Community Penalties*. Avebury, Aldershot.

Maluccio A. (1998) Assessing child welfare outcomes: the American perspective. *Children and Society*, **12**, 161–8.

Martinson R. (1974) What works? Questions and answers about prison reform. *Public Interest*, **35**, 405–17.

Mayer J. & Timms N. (1970) *The Client Speaks*. Routledge and Kegan Paul, London.

Mullen E.J. & Dumpson J.R. (1972) *Evaluation of Social Intervention*. Jossey-Bass, San Francisco.

Munro E. (1998) *Understanding Social Work: An Empirical Approach*. Athlone Press, London.

Oliver S. (1997) Lay perspectives on questions of effectiveness. In A. Maynard & I. Chalmers (eds) *Non-Random Reflections on Health Services Research*. BMJ Publishing Group, London.

Palmer T. (1995) Programmatic and non-programmatic aspects of successful intervention: new directions for research. *Crime and Delinquency*, **41**, 100–31.

Pannizon A., Olsen-Raymer G. & Guerra N. (1991) *Delinquency prevention: What Works, What Doesn't*. California Office of Criminal Justice Planning, Sacramento.

Parsloe P. & Stevenson O. (1978) *Social Service Teams: the Practitioners' View*. DHSS, London.

Parton N. (1996) Social work, risk and 'the blaming system'. In N. Parton (ed.) *Social Theory, Social Change and Social Work*. Routledge, London.

Pawson R. (1997) Evaluation methodology: back to basics. In G. Mair (ed.) *Evaluating the Effectiveness of Community Penalties*. Avebury, Aldershot.

Pecora P. (1997) *Examining the Effectiveness of Family Foster Care: a Select Literature Review*. The Casey Family Program, Seattle, WA.

Pincus A. & Minahan A. (1973) *Social Work Practice: Model and Method*. Peacock, Itasea, IL.

Powers E. & Witmer H. (1951) *An Experiment in the Prevention of Delinquency: the Cambridge–Somerville Youth Study*. Columbia University Press, New York.

Raynor P., Smith D. & Vanstone M. (1994) *Effective Probation Practice*. Macmillan, Basingstoke.

Reid W. & Hanrahan P. (1980) The effectiveness of social work: recent evidence. In E. Gordberg & N. Conrell (eds) *Evaluative Research in Social Care*. Heinemann, London.

Reid W. & Hanrahan P. (1982) Recent evaluations of social work: grounds for optimism. *Social Work*, **27**, 328–40.

Roberts C., Burnett R., Kirby A. & Hamill H. (1996) *A System for Evaluating Probation Practice. Probation Studies Unit Report No. 1*. Centre for Criminological Research, University of Oxford, Oxford.

Ross R. & Fabiano E. (1985) *Time to Think: a Cognitive Model of Delinquency Prevention and Rehabilitation*. Academy of Arts and Sciences, Johnson City.

Rowe J. & Lambert L. (1974) *Children Who Wait: A Study of Children Needing Substitute Families*. Association of British Adoption Agencies, London.

Rubin A. (1985) Practice effectiveness: more grounds for optimism. *Social Work*, **30**, 469–76.

Sainsbury E. (1975) *Social Work With Families: Perceptions of Social Casework Among Clients of a Family Service Unit*. RKP, London.

Secker J. (1993) *From Theory to Practice in Social Work*. Avebury, Aldershot.

Segal S. (1972) Research on the outcomes of social work therapeutic interventions: a review of the literature. *Journal of Health and Social Behaviour*, **13**, 3–17.

Sellick C. & Thoburn J. (1997) *What Works in Family Placement?* Barnardos, London.

Sheldon B. (1983) The use of single case experimental designs in the evaluation of social work effectiveness. *British Journal of Social Work*, **13**, 477–500.

Sheldon B. (1986) Social work effectiveness experiments: review and implications. *British Journal of Social Work*, **16**, 223–42.

Sinclair R. & Jacobs C. (1995) *Research in the Personal Social Services: the Experiences of Three Local Authorities*. National Children's Bureau, London.

Smith G. & Cantley C. (1985) *Assessing Health Care*. Open University Press, Buckingham.

Social Services Inspectorate (1993) *Evaluating Child Protection Services: Findings and Issues*. DoH, London.

Social Work Research Centre (1998) *Is Social Work Effective?* Social Work Research Centre, University of Stirling, Stirling.

Stationery Office (1998) *Modernising Social Services*. Cm 4169. Stationery Office, London.

Stein M. (1997) *What Works in Leaving Care?* Barnardos, London.

Thomlinson R. (1984) Something works: evidence from practice effectiveness studies. *Social Work*, **29**, 51–7.

Thyer B. & Thyer K. (1994) Single system research designs in social work practice: a bibliography from 1965 to 1990. *The Behavioural Social Work Review*, **15** (2), 5–12.

Trinder L. (1996) Social work research: the state of the art (or science). *Child and Family Social Work*, **1**, 233–42.

Tyson K. (1995) *New Foundations for Scientific Social and Behavioural Research*. Allyn & Bacon, Boston.

Underdown A. (1988) *Strategies for Effective Offender Supervision*. Home Office Inspectorate of Probation, London.

Videka-Sherman L. (1988) Meta-analysis of research on social work practice in mental health. *Social Work*, **33**, 325–38.

Walker H. & Beaumont B. (1981) *Probation Work: Critical Theory and Socialist Practice*. Blackwell, Oxford.

Webb D. (1996) Regulation for radicals: the state, CCETSW and the academy. In N. Parton (ed.) *Social Theory, Social Change and Social Work*. Routledge, London.

Whitehead J. & Lab S. (1989) A meta-analysis of juvenile correctional treatment. *Journal of Research in Crime and Delinquency*, **26**, 276–95.

Witkin S. (1996) If empirical practice is the answer, then what is the question? *Social Work Research*, **20**, 69–75.

Wood K.M. (1978) Casework effectiveness: a new look at the research evidence. *Social Work*, **23**, 437–59.

Chapter 8

Evidence-Based Practice in Education and the Contribution of Educational Research[1]

Martyn Hammersley

Introduction

There is some variation across fields in what a shift to evidence-based practice is believed to require. In medicine, most of the emphasis has been on the need for practitioners to make more use of research evidence in their work. In education, by contrast, the stress has been on the inadequacy of the research evidence that is available, as regards both rigour and applicability. In short, while the focus in medicine has been the quality of practice, in education it has been the quality of research. Thus, in late 1998 there were two officially sponsored reviews of educational research which were highly critical of it in these terms (Tooley 1998; Hillage *et al.* 1998). On the basis of these, the government drew up an action plan to resurrect educational research (see Clarke 1998).

It is only very recently that the term 'evidence-based practice' has appeared in the field of education. As yet, it has been used primarily in relation to school teaching, rather than to teaching in other contexts, or to educational administration and management. In the UK the Teacher Training Agency (TTA) has played a crucial role in this development, announcing its commitment to the promotion of teaching as a research-based profession (e.g. see TTA 1996). A central theme in its literature is that there is insufficient educational research that is focused on the classroom and that supplies practical knowledge which can be used to improve the quality of teaching. In an attempt to correct this, the TTA has mounted a research programme designed to encourage such research on the part of teachers (for a review of the first fruits of this work, see Foster 1998).

It should be noted that, while use of the term evidence-based practice is relatively new, the idea that teaching ought to be based on research evidence has a long history (e.g. Dunkin & Biddle 1974). One of the pre-occupations of much American educational research in the first half of the twentieth century, and of later research in the UK, was the relative effectiveness of different pedagogical techniques and styles. The most common view among educational researchers today is that this project failed, not just for contingent reasons, but because it was mistaken in principle (Chambers 1992; Glass 1994; also Gage 1985, 1994). As a result, over the past few decades the role of research has come to be seen by many educational researchers more in terms of the enlightenment than the engineering model (Janowitz 1972; Bulmer 1982; Finch 1986). Rather than supplying or validating effective techniques or policies, the pay-off of research is now widely believed to lie more in terms of raising questions about current assumptions and of supplying alternative perspectives on the practice of teachers, education managers, and policy-makers, and on the situations in which they work.

Advocacy of teacher research, another component of the TTA project, is also far from new. There was an influential classroom action research movement in the US during the 1950s (Corey 1953), and in the UK and elsewhere from the 1970s onwards (Stenhouse 1975; Nixon 1981; Hustler *et al.* 1986; Elliott 1991). Moreover, these developments have also been subjected to critical assessment. Questions have been raised about whether such work is an adequate substitute for more conventional kinds of research, and about the contribution of some versions of it to classroom practice and to educational change (see Wiles 1953; Hodgkinson 1957; Carr & Kemmis 1986; Hammersley 1993).

Recent advocacy of evidence-based teaching in the UK has not drawn much on this past experience, the proposal being presented instead as a radically new venture. Furthermore, it has occurred in a context where, as in the public sector generally, there has been growing emphasis on so-called transparent public accountability, framed in terms of attempts to measure the value added by institutional practice. From this point of view, research is often seen as playing a crucial role in providing the means by which to monitor the inputs, processes, and outputs of institutions, and in offering guidance about how best to render services more effective and efficient. It is against this background that educational research has been criticised as inadequate.

By far the most considered and effective presentation of the case for the failure of educational research to facilitate evidence-based teaching is to be found in David Hargreaves' TTA lecture 'Teaching as a Research-based Profession' (Hargreaves 1996). The rest of this chapter will outline his arguments and assess them.

Hargreaves' TTA lecture

Hargreaves argues that the effectiveness of teaching in schools would be substantially improved if it were a research-based profession. And he lays the blame for the fact that it is not on researchers rather than on teachers. He argues that current educational research is neither sufficiently cumulative nor sufficiently relevant to teachers' practical concerns for it to make the contribution required of it. To support his argument, Hargreaves draws a contrast between the role of research in education and its contribution to the practice of medicine, using evidence-based medicine as a model.

His first criticism of educational research is that much of it is non-cumulative, in the sense that it does not explicitly 'build on earlier research – by confirming or falsifying it, by extending or refining it, by replacing it with better evidence or theory, and so on' (Hargreaves 1996: 1). The problem is that 'a few small-scale investigations of an issue which are never followed up inevitably produce inconclusive and contestable findings of little practical relevance'. Moreover, replications, 'which are more necessary in the social than the natural sciences because of the importance of contextual and cultural variations, are astonishingly rare'. This situation is worsened by the fact that 'educational researchers, like other social scientists, are often engaged in bitter disputes among themselves about the philosophy and methodology of the social sciences'. This means that lines of research are abandoned when there is a change in fashion, rather than because problems have been solved. As a result, despite considerable work, 'there are few areas which have yielded a corpus of research evidence regarded as scientifically sound and as a worthwhile resource to guide professional action' (Hargreaves 1996: 2).

This first argument leads straight into the second: that research is not found useful by teachers. Hargreaves claims that 'few successful practising teachers' use the knowledge provided by the foundation disciplines (psychology, sociology, philosophy, and history) or think it important for their practice. Indeed, 'teachers are able to be effective in their work in almost total ignorance of this infrastructure' (Hargreaves 1996). As a result:

> 'the disciplines of education are seen to consist of "theory" which is strongly separated from practice. Trainee teachers soon spot the yawning gap between theory and practice and the low value of research as a guide to the solution of practical problems'.
>
> (Hargreaves 1996: 2)

The fundamental defect, then, is that there is no substantial body of research 'which, if only it were disseminated and acted on by teachers, would yield huge benefits in the quality of teaching and learning' (Hargreaves 1996). To underline the point, Hargreaves asks: 'just how much research is there which: (i) demonstrates conclusively that if teachers change their practice from x to y there will be a significant and enduring improvement in teaching and learning; and (ii) has developed an effective method of convincing teachers of the benefits of, and means to, changing from x to y' (Hargreaves 1996).

On the basis of his critique of educational research, Hargreaves argues that the money allocated to it is not well spent: 'Something has indeed gone badly wrong. Research is having little impact on the improvement of practice, and teachers I talk to do not think they get value for money from the £50–60 million we spend annually on educational research' (Hargreaves 1996: 5). He concludes from this that radical changes are required in the way that research is organised and carried out. In particular, 'practitioners and policy makers must take an active role in shaping the direction of educational research' (Hargreaves 1996: 6). He proposes the establishment of a national education research forum to facilitate dialogue amongst the various stakeholders. This would sponsor research foresight exercises to provide the basis for a national strategy, specifying short- and long-term priorities. He recommends the reallocation to the TTA and OFSTED (Office for Standards in Education) of some of the money currently given to universities for educational research. Above all, he argues that more research should be carried out by practising teachers, since this would enhance its practical relevance.

In the remainder of this chapter, I will examine each of Hargreaves' two main arguments about the failings of research in the field of education, before going on to examine his reliance on the medical analogy.

Educational research as non-cumulative

There is some force in Hargreaves' argument here. Commitment to one-off studies is a defect of much educational research, and indeed of social research generally. It reduces the extent to which findings from particular investigations are tested across different situations and minimises the division of labour, thereby undermining the cumulation of knowledge. There is little doubt, in my view, of the need to move to a situation where new research builds more effectively on earlier work, and where greater attention is given to testing competing interpretations of data, whether descriptive or explanatory. And this may require replications; though the form these take cannot be the same in naturalistic as in experimental research.

At the same time, there are also serious problems with this aspect of Hargreaves' critique of educational research. One is that he is not clear about what criteria he is using to assess the quality of that research. In the early parts of his lecture he stresses its failure to accumulate knowledge by building on earlier work, but the concept of cumulation is not a simple one: there are different forms it can take (see Freese 1980: 40–49). Moreover, there are educational researchers who claim that their work has produced theoretical development (see Woods 1985, 1987); Hargreaves does not make clear why he denies these claims – though in my view he is right to deny them (see Hammersley 1987a,b).

Later in his lecture, this first criticism turns into the charge that educational research itself is not, or that not enough of it is, evidence-based (Hargreaves 1996: 7). Again, clarification is required. What is and is not being accepted as evidence here, and what counts as basing claims on evidence? This is an issue which stands out sharply in the context of the comparison between research on medicine and education. The evidence-based medicine movement takes the randomised controlled trial (RCT) as the ideal source of evidence. It is much less clear what Hargreaves' ideal is, though there are indications that it is experimental research. However, he does not explicitly defend that ideal, in a field in which its value and feasibility have been seriously questioned.

A second, and related point is that Hargreaves presents the failings of current educational research as if they stemmed solely from a lack of commitment on the part of researchers to rigorous and cumulative enquiry. There is no doubt that this commitment has become attenuated. But, to some extent, this is a response to genuine difficulties. As Hargreaves knows, since he was a leading figure in it, the shift to qualitative methods among educational researchers in the 1970s was prompted by powerful criticisms identifying unresolved problems in earlier quantitative research. Some of these related to the difficulties of measuring what is of educational significance (Delamont & Hamilton 1984; Barrow 1984). Others concerned the peculiar complexities of 'social causation', including interaction effects (Cronbach 1975). The most radical versions of these arguments drew on philosophical writings to the effect that human social life is quite different in character from the physical world studied by natural scientists (and, we might add, from that investigated by most medical researchers) (see Winch 1958; Schutz 1967). From this it was often concluded that the kind of knowledge produced by natural scientists is not available to social and educational researchers.

While the arguments for the distinctiveness of the social world may have been overplayed, there can be no denying the serious problems involved in producing conclusive knowledge about causal patterns in social phenomena. This is one reason why educational researchers, like social scientists generally, have become embroiled in philosophical and methodological disputes. Hargreaves treats these disputes as if they were merely a matter of fashion. But, while some of the discussion may be self-indulgent, the underlying problems are real enough. At their core is precisely the question of the extent to which one can have a science of human behaviour of a kind that models itself, even remotely, on the natural sciences. By failing to mention these problems, Hargreaves implies that the sort of cumulative, well-founded knowledge he wants can be created simply by researchers pulling themselves together and getting back to work (under the direction of teachers). The problem is not so simple, and not so easily remedied.

The difficulties faced by educational research can only be sketched briefly here. As already noted, they centre on two areas: the measurement of social phenomena and the validation of causal relationships amongst those phenomena. As regards the former, there are problems involved in identifying distinct and standardised 'treatments' in education, witness the difficulties encountered by researchers seeking to distinguish teaching styles (see Bennett 1976; Wragg 1976; Galton *et al.* 1980). Indeed, there are unresolved measurement problems even in relation to the most specific and concrete aspects of teaching, for example types of questions asked (Scarth & Hammersley 1986a,b). The problems are also formidable at the other end of the causal chain, in operationalising the concept of learning. There is room for considerable disagreement about what students should learn, as well as about what they actually learn, in any particular situation in terms of: different knowledge, skills, and/or values; depth versus sur- face learning; degrees of transferability and so on. More than this, very often what are regarded as the most important kinds of learning – relating to high-level, transferable cognitive skills or personal understanding – are extraordinarily difficult to measure with any degree of validity and reli- ability, and there are doubts about whether replicable measurement of them is possible, even in principle. In short, in both areas, there are ques- tions about whether it is possible to move beyond 'sensitising' concepts to the definitive concepts that seem to be required for scientific analysis of the kind proposed by Hargreaves.

The problems relating to the establishment of causal patterns are equally severe. Since we are interested in what goes on in real schools and colleges, and because strict experimentation is often ruled out for practical or ethical reasons, this task becomes extremely difficult. How are we to control competing factors in such a way as to assess the relative contribution of each one in what is usually a complex web of relationships? More than this, can we assume that causation in this field involves fixed, universal relationships, rather than local context-sensitive patterns in which inter- pretation and decision on the part of teachers and students play an important role? Unlike most areas of medicine, in education the treatments consist of symbolic interaction, with all the scope for multiple interpreta- tions and responses which that implies. What kind of causal relations are involved here, if they are causal at all? And what kind of knowledge can we have of them?

These are, then, some of the fundamental problems facing educational researchers attempting to produce the kind of knowledge that Hargreaves demands. I do not want to suggest that such knowledge is impossible, but he seems greatly to underestimate the difficulties.

There is another point too. In my view, one important cause of the unsatisfactory nature of much educational research is that it is too pre- occupied with producing information that will shape *current* policy or practice. This seems likely to be one source of the lack of testing and cumulation of knowledge that Hargreaves complains about. He touches on this when he notes that educational researchers have fallen between two stools: 'achieving neither prestige from the social scientists . . . nor gratitude from classroom teachers' (Hargreaves 1996: 3). The problem, in part, is that while working under the aegis of academic disciplines concerned with contributing to theory, researchers have also sought to address the changing political agendas that define pressing educational problems. This is partly a product of sharp competition for funding. But it has also been encouraged by conceptions of research which imply that it is possible simultaneously to contribute to scientific theory and to provide solutions to practical or political problems. This view is characteristic of some forms of action research, including Lewin's version, to which Hargreaves is sympathetic.

In my judgement, though, this assumption of the unity of theory and practice is fallacious, since the production of information of high practical relevance usually depends on a great deal of knowledge that does not have such immediate relevance. In other words, for science to be able to contribute knowledge that is relevant to practice, a division of labour is required: a great deal of coordinated work is necessary tackling smaller, more manageable problems that do not have direct pay-off. Moreover, this requires sustained work over a long period, not short bursts of activity geared to political and practical priorities. In other words, the wrong time-schedule has prevailed in much educational enquiry: that of educational policy-making and practice, rather than that appropriate to true scientific research.

In effect, then, the commitment of educational researchers to addressing the big questions and to producing answers to them in the short rather than the long term, along with parallel expectations on the part of funders, has been a major contributing factor to the weaknesses that Hargreaves identifies. His call for educational research to be more practically effective will only worsen this problem. He insists that 'curiosity-driven, long-term "basic" and "blue skies" research is as vital in education as in any other scientific field' (Hargreaves 1996: 7). But he neglects the extent to which the funding for this has already been eroded. For example, the main source which he mentions, the ESRC (the Economic and Social Research Council), has increasingly moved towards non-responsive funding, to an emphasis on strategic and even applied research. This is despite the fact that its predecessor, the SSRC (Social Sciences Research Council), was specifically established to fund basic research – government departments and other sources were expected to finance applied work. Moreover, Hargreaves applauds 'the pressure the ESRC now puts on researchers to demonstrate consultation with, and involvement of, users as a condition of getting a research grant' (Hargreaves 1996: 6). Yet it is a feature of basic research that who the users will be and what use they might make of it are largely unknown.

Contributing to practice

As we saw, Hargreaves' second theme was that educational research has not produced sufficient practically relevant knowledge. Few researchers are likely to deny that an important ultimate aim of all research should be to produce knowledge which has practical relevance. But there is room for much disagreement about what such relevance amounts to, and about what kinds of knowledge are possible and of value. In his lecture, Hargreaves adopts a narrowly instrumental view: that research should be able to tell practitioners which is the best technique for dealing with a particular kind of problem. In other words, research is portrayed as directed towards finding or evaluating solutions to technical problems.

Questions about whether educational research can supply the sort of knowledge demanded by this instrumentalist view have already been raised in the previous section, but there is also the issue of whether the problems that teachers face are of a kind that is open to solution by research; in other words, whether they are technical in character. Early on in his lecture, Hargreaves seems to recognise that they may not be. He comments:

'both education and medicine are profoundly people-centred professions. Neither believes that helping people is merely a matter of a simple and technical application but rather a highly skilled process in which a sophisticated judgement matches a professional decision to the unique needs of each client'.

(Hargreaves 1996: 1)

However, his subsequent discussion of the contribution which he would like to see research making to educational practice seems to contradict this; for example, his reference to research needing to 'demonstrate conclusively' that a particular pedagogical approach will produce 'a significant and enduring improvement' (Hargreaves 1996: 5).

As I noted at the beginning of this chapter, at one time it was widely assumed that educational practice could, and should, be based on scientific theory, with teachers using techniques whose appropriateness had been determined by the results of scientific investigation. However, much recent work on the nature of teaching by philosophers, psychologists, and sociologists has emphasised the extent to which it is practical rather than technical in character; in brief, that it is a matter of making judgements rather than following rules (Schwab 1969; Hirst 1983; Carr 1987; Olson 1992). This line of argument throws doubt on the idea that teaching can be *based* on research knowledge. It implies that it necessarily depends on experience, wisdom, local knowledge, and judgement. And it seems likely that it is precisely the practical character of teaching, as much as any failing on the part of researchers, which is the main source of the yawning gap between theory and practice that Hargreaves bemoans; witness the fact that complaints about such gaps are a commonplace of professional education in all fields (see Schön 1983, 1987).

One of the features of much practical activity, and particularly of teaching, is that goals are multiple, and their meaning is open to dispute and is difficult to operationalise. In this context, Hargreaves' focus on the 'effectiveness' of pedagogy obscures some of the most important issues. Put into practice, an exclusive focus on effectiveness leads to an over-emphasis on those outcomes which can be measured, at the expense of other educational goals. We see this problem in currently influential research on school effectiveness. While researchers in this field are usually careful to note that the outcome measures they use do not exhaust or measure all the goals of schooling, their work is sometimes presented and often interpreted as measuring school effectiveness *as such* (see Elliott 1996; Sammons & Reynolds 1997).

Of course, we need to take care not to adopt too sharp a distinction between technical and practical activities. What is involved is more of a continuum, and it seems likely that educational practice is not homogeneous in this respect: there may be some educational problems that are open to technical solution, even though many are not. Nevertheless, in general terms, all teaching beyond that concerned with very elementary skills seems likely to come closer to the practical end of the dimension. And the practical character of most teachers' work is increased by the fact that they deal with batches of pupils, rather than with single clients, as in the case of medicine. It is this which makes the classroom situation a particularly demanding one in terms of the need for reliance on contextual judgement (Jackson 1968; Doyle 1977).

All this is certainly not to suggest that research can make no contribution to teaching. But it means that the contribution cannot take the form of indicating which is the appropriate technique to use in a particular situation, or even what are the chances of success using a particular technique in given types of situation. The nature of the contribution is more likely to involve the provision of information that corrects assumptions or alters the context in which teachers view some aspect of their situation, for example by highlighting possible causal relations to which they may not routinely give attention. Equally important is the capacity that research has for illuminating aspects of teachers' practice that are below the normal level of their consciousness. A good example of this is research on teachers' typifications of children. Documentation of how these are built up, how they affect the ways in which teachers deal with pupils, and the consequences of this, is surely of considerable value (see Hargreaves *et al.* 1975). For the most part, such contributions are not dramatic in their consequences. But it is just as much a mistake to try to judge the value of research in terms of its immediate and identifiable practical impact as it is to judge the quality of a school solely by its examination results.

All this raises questions about Hargreaves' judgement that educational research does not offer value for money. This phrase has become a popular one, but it involves a judgement that is a good deal more complex and uncertain than is generally recognised. Hargreaves gives no indication of how he thinks the cost–benefit analysis involved could be carried out. Even measuring the real cost of a particular piece of research would be a for-midable task, and measuring the value of its impact would be virtually impossible and always open to debate. Nor does he acknowledge the problems with the whole cost–benefit approach. These have long been recognised within economics, if not always given the weight they deserve (see Little 1950). Because of their reliance on values, all judgements about cost-effectiveness are likely to be subject to considerable instability across time, circumstances and observers. So the question arises of who is to judge, when, and how. For the purposes of his lecture, Hargreaves relies most explicitly on the judgements of teachers he has talked with (Hargreaves 1996: 5). Even apart from the sampling and reactivity problems involved here, we can ask whether teachers are the best judges, given that according to Hargreaves they have little knowledge of the findings of educational research. Furthermore, teachers are not the only proper audi-ence for such research. Its main function, surely, is to inform public debates about educational issues: to provide information for use by anyone con-cerned with those issues, not only teachers but also parents, governors, administrators, pressure groups, politicians and citizens generally. How well it does this is an important question, and some assessment of its cost-effectiveness in this respect may be unavoidable; but this can be no more than a speculative and contestable estimate, and should be labelled as such.

The parallel with medicine

In his critique of the practical failure of educational research, Hargreaves relies heavily on the analogy with medicine. However, as with all analo-gies, it is important to recognise that there may be significant differences, as well as similarities, between what is being compared. Also, analogies are sometimes based on misconceptions about the comparative standard being used. We ought to be very cautious, then, about using the case of medicine as a basis for evaluating educational research and practice. Its appro-priateness has to be argued for, not assumed.

In the previous two sections I have discussed aspects of the field of education which make it different from that of medicine, in ways that challenge Hargreaves' negative judgements about the relative success of educational research. Certainly, it seems likely that much medical research avoids many of the problems that face educational researchers, in particular those deriving from the peculiarities of the social world. Where it does not, I suggest, we find the same lack of cumulative evidence that Hargreaves complains about in education. Similarly, medical practice may generally be closer to the technical rather than to the practical end of the spectrum, so that research is often able to play a role there which is much closer to that envisaged by the 'engineering' model than is possible in education.

At the same time, there are respects in which the assumptions Hargreaves makes about medical research, and about the way it contributes to medical practice, are open to doubt. One concerns the contrast in quality that he draws between medical and educational research. It is of note that rather similar criticisms to those he levelled at educational research have been directed at medical research carried out by doctors (see Anderson 1990; Feussner 1996). In an article entitled *The scandal of poor medical research*, Altman comments:

> 'When I tell friends outside medicine that many papers published in medical journals are misleading because of methodological weaknesses they are rightly shocked. Huge sums of money are spent annually on research that is seriously flawed through use of inappropriate designs, unrepresentative samples, small samples, incorrect methods of analysis, and faulty interpretation'.
>
> (Altman 1994: 283)

It is worth emphasising the reasons that Altman puts forward for the poor quality of much medical research, since these relate directly to what Hargreaves claims to be its great strength: the fact that it is carried out by practising doctors. Altman lays the blame on the fact that doctors are expected to engage in research, but are often inadequately prepared for or committed to it. What we may conclude from this is that while there is undoubtedly a great deal more cumulation of well-founded knowledge in medicine than in education, it is not at all clear that this results primarily from the participation of clinicians. On this basis we might reasonably fear that increasing the proportion of educational research that is carried out by practising teachers would not provide a remedy for the methodological ills that Hargreaves has identified.

There are also questions about the assumptions which Hargreaves makes about medical *practice*. Sociological research investigating this has highlighted the role of clinical judgement, and pointed to the emphasis that clinicians themselves place on it (Becker *et al.* 1961: 231–8; Freidson 1970). Thus, Becker *et al.* argue that clinical experience 'can be used to legitimate a choice of procedures for a patient's treatment and can even be used to rule out use of some procedures that have been scientifically established'

(Becker *et al.* 1961: 231). Similarly, Atkinson describes the clinician as 'essentially a pragmatist, relying on results rather than theory, and trusting in personal, first-hand knowledge rather than on abstract principles or "book knowledge"' (Atkinson 1981: 5). In a more recent study of hematologists, he shows how personal, traditional and scientific knowledge interpenetrate even in clinical discourse away from the bedside (Atkinson 1995: 48 ff).

Two closely related aspects of the picture of clinical practice presented by this research are relevant here. First, clinical decision-making is not based solely, or even primarily, on knowledge drawn directly from research publications. Second, it often does not conform to what we might call the rationalistic model of medical procedure. According to this model, practice takes the following form: the relevant problem is clearly identified at the start; the full range of possible strategies for dealing with it are assessed in terms of their costs and benefits, on the basis of the best available evidence; and, finally, that strategy is selected and implemented which promises to be the most effective. As has been pointed out in many fields, including economics, for a variety of reasons practical activity deviates substantially from this rationalistic model: goals are not always clearly formulated and undergo change over the course of the activity; only a limited range of strategies may be considered, with little search for information about alternative strategies, stock assumptions being relied on; and the aim may not be to maximise pay-off but only to achieve a satisfactory solution, with scope for disagreement about what this amounts to (see Simon 1955; March 1988).

In one way, Hargreaves recognises these features of medical practice. Referring to some of Caroline Cox's comments about teachers, he points out how medical practitioners also often rely on 'tradition, prejudice, dogma, and ideology' (Hargreaves 1996: 7–8). In adopting this loaded characterisation, he aligns himself with the proponents of evidence-based medicine, who argue that research must play an increased role in clinical practice if the latter's effectiveness is to reach acceptable levels. They argue that there are reasons to doubt the effectiveness of a substantial proportion of medical treatments currently used by clinicians. Advocates of evidence-based medicine put forward two main explanations for this. First, they claim that the quality of clinical practice deteriorates over the course of practitioners' careers. This is because they are dependent on the state of research knowledge when they trained, which becomes progressively outmoded. The second argument is that the huge number of medical research reports now produced is too great for clinicians to access directly. What is required, therefore, is the use of bibliographical strategies and technology for summarising and making available the information produced by research, and the training of clinicians in the use of these.

What does not come through in Hargreaves' lecture is that evidence-based medicine is by no means an uncontroversial matter (see *The Lancet* 1995; Grahame-Smith 1995; Court 1996; and letters in *The Lancet* 1995, 1996). Critics have argued that it places too much emphasis on the role of research findings in clinical decision-making; in fact, that it is a misnomer, since all medicine is evidence-based, even when it does not make the kind of systematic use of the research literature that advocates of evidence-based medicine recommend. One critic points out that it would be better referred to as 'literature-based medicine' (Horwitz, cited in Shuchman 1996: 1396). Another suggests that the presumption built into the term is that the practice of medicine 'was previously based on a direct communication with God or the tossing of a coin' (Fowler 1995: 838). What is at issue is not the use of evidence as against reliance on something else (tradition, prejudice, dogma, and ideology), *but the relative importance of different kinds of evidence*. And we should perhaps also note that the appropriate balance amongst these will vary not just across medical specialties but also at different stages of treatment. In diagnosis, for example, particular emphasis is likely to be given to evidence from medical histories, physical examinations and/or test results.

Critics also point out some problems in the use of research evidence to inform clinical decision-making. One is that the literature is very variable in quality, and that there is much more research in some areas than others. A consequence of this is that there are significant gaps in reliable knowledge which render the practice of evidence-based medicine problematic in many fields. More significantly, the fact that there may be evidence about some treatments and not others, or better evidence about them, could enable misleading conclusions to be drawn about their relative efficacy. A second point is that there may be biases in the research literature, for example resulting from the tendency of journals to be less interested in publishing negative than positive findings. A third problem is that the process of summarising the findings and methods of research may itself introduce distortions. Certainly, it makes the critical appraisal of evidence, which advocates of evidence-based medicine emphasise, more difficult and subject to increased threats to validity.

There are also problems surrounding the *application* of information about aggregates to particular patients. The authors of a key text in clinical epidemiology, one of the foundations of evidence-based medicine, report a senior doctor as opining that it is immoral to combine epidemiology with clinical practice (Sackett *et al.* 1985). It is not clear from the context what the reasoning was behind this criticism, but two problems seem relevant. One is that there may be circumstances where the requirements of research conflict with those of treating a particular patient. An illustration is provided by Jadad (1996), in an article entitled 'Are you playing evidence-based medicine games with our daughter?' He seems to have fed his three-and-a-half-year-old daughter shrimp in order to test a consultant's diagnosis of allergy, which he believed was not based on sound research evidence. Whatever the rights and wrongs of this particular case, it is not difficult to see that conflicting motivations can be involved where clinicians (or parents!) are also engaged in research (see also Dearlove *et al.* 1995: 258).

Another issue relates to the problem of treating a patient as a category for which one has research data. Clinicians are directly responsible for the treatment of individual patients, not primarily concerned with what works *in general*. Patients always have multiple characteristics, some of which may be such as to render the treatment indicated by the research literature inappropriate; and these characteristics can include patients' preferences (see Thornton 1992; Charlton 1995: 257; Jones & Sagar 1995: 258).

Even putting aside the problem of applying aggregate data to individual cases, it is not necessarily in a patient's best interests for a clinician to use what is reported in the literature as the most effective treatment. Treatments can demand considerable skills, which a particular practitioner may not have, most obviously (but not exclusively) in the case of surgery. Thus, what is in evidential terms a 'less effective' treatment, but one in which the doctor already has experience, may be more advantageous than a less-than-fully-successful attempt at something more ambitious (see Burkett & Knafl 1974: 94–5). Literature-based knowledge can only provide a guide; it is no substitute for first-hand experience, or for discussion with immediate colleagues who can be questioned further in the event of unforeseen outcomes. Thus, a particular technique may be used because it seems to have been effective in the past, and also because much is known about what to expect from it: one knows what normally happens as well as the routine deviance associated with it. Using new drugs or surgical techniques can increase the level of uncertainty, and the danger of running into unforeseen situations outside one's experience.

It seems unlikely that any clinician would deny the value of research evidence. What is at issue is the degree and nature of its use. The advocates of evidence-based medicine vary in what they recommend. Sometimes, they simply point to the capacity for searching the research literature that is now provided by information management technology; emphasising that this cannot substitute for experience and clinical judgement. On other occasions, however, more radical proposals seem to be implied, where systematic literature searches are treated as obligatory and as providing benefit : risk ratios which can form the basis not just for clinical decision-making but also for accountability. In this, advocates of evidence-based medicine follow Cochrane's dismissal of clinical *opinion*, and his argument that there is little or no evidence about the effectiveness of many routinely used techniques, where evidence is interpreted as the outcome of RCTs or as 'immediate and obvious' effects (Cochrane 1972: 30). What is at issue here, then, is not just what is, and is not, to count as adequate evidence, but also the approach to be adopted in clinical decision-making, how it is to be assessed, and by whom.

Sociologists have often noted the role that an emphasis on clinical judgement plays in the power that the medical profession exercises. Evidence-based medicine threatens this power, since it meshes with demands for doctors to be more externally accountable, not just in terms of efficacy but also of cost-effectiveness. It is this which has caused a reaction against evidence-based practice in some parts of the medical community. But it would only be justifiable to dismiss this resistance as ingrained conservatism, or self-interested concern with preserving professional power, if there were good reasons to be confident that research evidence could replace clinical judgement, and that the rationalistic model could be applied. Yet there seem to be few grounds for confidence about this, even though moves towards clearer guidelines for clinicians and increased use of medical research findings may well be desirable.

As in the NHS, so also in the education system there has been growing emphasis on transparent public accountability and attempts to set up quasi-markets which maximise efficiency. Moreover, Hargreaves clearly has this kind of accountability very much in mind when he argues that:

> 'expertise *means* not just having relevant experience and knowledge but having *demonstrable* competence and clear *evidence* to justify doing things in one way rather than another'.
>
> (Hargreaves 1996: 7)

And this is very much in line with the policy of the TTA (see Millett 1996). From this point of view, a research-based teaching profession is one that accounts for itself in terms of the details of its practice to those outside by appeal to the following of explicitly formulated procedures backed by research evidence.

Just as evidence-based medicine threatens to assist attacks on the professionalism of doctors by managers in the NHS, so evidence-based practice in education seems to be a formula designed to render teachers more transparently accountable. In both areas there are grave doubts about whether this will improve quality of service. It seems at least as likely further to demoralise and undermine the professional judgement of practitioners, in occupations that have already been seriously damaged in these respects.

Conclusion

In this chapter, looking at the recent emergence of calls for evidence-based practice in education, I have examined David Hargreaves' arguments about the failure of educational research to provide a foundation for this: its failure to supply a cumulated body of sound knowledge about the effectiveness and efficiency of different pedagogic techniques. Hargreaves' lecture raises very important issues, and some of his criticisms of educational research are telling. Researchers probably do need to be more focused about what their goals are, and more concerned about the degree of success they have had in achieving them, and about the problems they face. Furthermore, it is necessary to make research both build more effectively on earlier work and provide a better foundation for subsequent investigations.

At the same time, there are some fundamental defects in Hargreaves' analysis. One is that he is not very explicit about the form he believes educational research should take, and in terms of this he evaluates current work negatively. Another is his neglect of the severe methodological problems that educational researchers face. Hargreaves seems to see the task of developing cumulative knowledge about the effectiveness of different pedagogical techniques as much more straightforward than it is. Here, as elsewhere, his reliance on the medical analogy is potentially misleading. Much medical research, while by no means easy or unproblematic, does not involve the distinctive problems associated with studying social phenomena. We might also note that while Hargreaves stresses the amount of money spent on educational research, this is only a tiny fraction of that allocated to medical research (for which he provides no estimate). Like is not being compared with like here, in either respect.

Another problem concerns the nature of the relationship that is possible between research and practice in the field of education. I have argued that Hargreaves uses a standard to judge current educational research which assumes too direct and instrumental a form of that relationship. Even in the field of medicine, it is not clear that this model can be closely approximated. And the throughly practical character of teaching – the diverse and difficult-to-operationalise goals, the multiple variables and complex relationships involved – may mean that research can rarely provide sound information about the relative effectiveness of different techniques which is directly applicable. The history of research on effective teaching points strongly in this direction. Furthermore, in my view there is a tension between seeking to improve the rigour of educational enquiry so as to contribute to the cumulation of knowledge, on the one hand, and trying to make its findings have more direct practical relevance, on the other. There are, of course, those who see no tension here at all; but Hargreaves does not make a case for this, and the history of action research, in education and elsewhere, suggests a tension between these two views (see Rapoport 1970).

Hargreaves' prescriptions should not be rejected entirely. Practical research carried out by teachers and educational managers in order to further their work can be useful; so long as it is recognised that not every problem needs research to find a solution, and that many practically relevant questions cannot be answered by research, at least not within the time-frame required. However, there are dangers in this kind of work being required to meet a scientific canon, since it is designed to serve a different purpose. While there will be some overlap in techniques and relevant considerations between academic and practical research, the goals should be different. Practical enquiries are no substitute for academic research; just as the latter is no substitute for them.

Finally, what Hargreaves recommends involves a transformation of teaching as well as of research, even though he gives much less emphasis to this. In particular, it involves extending the accountability of teachers beyond examination league tables and national tests, to the requirement that they justify the details of classroom practice in terms of research evidence. And this seems likely to undermine professionalism rather than to promote it.

Advocates of evidence-based medicine have often been challenged because they are not able to support their proposals with the kind of evidence that they demand of medical practitioners (see Norman 1995). Hargreaves and the TTA are also vulnerable to this kind of charge, especially given the radical nature of the treatment proposed in relation to both research and teaching. Hargreaves certainly does not provide evidence which 'demonstrates conclusively that if [researchers] change their practice from x to y there will be a significant and enduring improvement in teaching and learning' (Hargreaves 1996: 4). Given the absence of this evidence, we must conclude that the remedies proposed are at least as likely to worsen the problems faced by educational researchers and teachers as they are to provide a cure.

Notes

1. This is a shortened and modified version of a paper written for the *British Educational Research Journal* (Hammersley 1996). David Hargreaves wrote a rejoinder to it (Hargreaves 1997), and a reply to this is available from the author (Hammersley 1997). My thanks to Roger Gomm for discussion of the ideas in this paper; and also to Paul Atkinson, Richard Edwards and Donald Mackinnon for comments on an earlier version.

References

Altman D.G. (1994) The scandal of poor medical research. *British Medical Journal,* **308**, 283–4.

Anderson B. (1990) *Methodological Errors in Medical Research.* Blackwell, Oxford.

Atkinson P.A. (1981) *The Clinical Experience.* Gower, Farnborough.

Atkinson P.A. (1995) *Medical Talk and Medical Work.* Sage, London.

Barrow R. (1984) *Giving Teaching Back to Teachers.* Wheatsheaf, Brighton.

Becker H.S., Geer B., Hughes E.C. & Strauss A. (1961) *Boys in White: Student Culture in Medical School.* Chicago University Press, Chicago.

Bennett N. (1976) *Teaching Styles and Pupil Progress.* Open Books, London.

Bulmer M. (1982) *The Uses of Social Research.* Allen and Unwin, London.

Burkett G. & Knafl K. (1974) Judgement and decision-making in a medical speciality. *Sociology of Work and Occupations,* **1**, 82–109.

Carr W. (1987) What is an educational practice? *Journal of the Philosophy of Education,* **21**, 163–75.

Carr W. & Kemmis S. (1986) *Becoming Critical.* Falmer, Lewes.

Chambers J.H. (1992) *Empiricist Research on Teaching: a Philosophical and Practical Critique of its Scientific Pretensions.* Kluwer, Boston.

Charlton B. (1995) Megatrials are subordinate to medical science. *British Medical Journal,* **311**, 257.

Clancy C. (1996) Evidence-based medicine meets cost-effectiveness analysis (editorial). *Journal of the American Medical Association,* **276**, 329–30.

Clarke C. (1998) Resurrecting research to raise standards. *Social Sciences,* **39**, October 2. Economic and Social Research Council, Swindon.

Cochrane A.L. (1972) *Effectiveness and Efficiency.* Nuffield Provincial Hospitals Trust, Oxford.

Corey S. (1953) *Action Research to Improve School Practices.* Teachers' College, Columbia University, New York.

Court C. (1996) NHS Handbook criticises evidence-based medicine. *British Medical Journal,* **312**, 1439–40.

Cronbach L. (1975) Beyond the two disciplines of scientific psychology. *American Psychologist,* **30**, 116–27.

Dearlove O, Sharples A., O'Brien K. & Dunkley C. (1995) Many questions cannot be answered by evidence based-medicine. *British Medical Journal,* **311**, 257–8.

Delamont S. & Hamilton D. (1984) Revisiting classroom research: a continuing cautionary tale. In S. Delamont (ed.) *Readings on Interaction in the Classroom.* Methuen, London.

Doyle W. (1977) Learning the classroom environment. *Journal of Teacher Education,* **28**, 51–5.

Dunkin M.J. & Biddle B.J. (1974) *The Study of Teaching.* Holt, Rinehart & Winston, New York.

Elliott J. (1991) *Action Research for Educational Change.* Open University Press, Milton Keynes.

Elliott J. (1996) School effectiveness research and its critics: alternative visions of schooling. *Cambridge Journal of Education,* **26**, 199–224.

Feussner J. (1996) Evidence-based medicine: new priority for an old paradigm. *Journal of Bone and Mineral Research,* **11**, 877–82.

Finch J. (1986) *Research and Policy: the Uses of Qualitative Methods in Social and Education Research.* Falmer, Lewes.

Foster P. (1998) '*Never mind the quality, feel the impact': some critical comments on the TTA Teacher Research Pilot Scheme,* unpublished.

Foster P., Gomm R. & Hammersley M. (1996) *Constructing Educational Inequality: an Assessment of Research on School Processes.* Falmer, London.

Fowler P.B.S. (1995) Letter. *Lancet*, **346**, 838.

Freese L. (1980) The problem of cumulative knowledge. In I. Freese (ed.) *Theoretical Methods in Sociology*. University of Pittsburgh Press, Pittsburgh.

Freidson E. (1970) *Profession of Medicine: a Study of the Sociology of Applied Knowledge*. Dodd, Mead & Co., New York.

Gage N.L. (1985) *Hard Gains in the Soft Sciences: the Case of Pedagogy*. Phi Delta Kappa, Bloomington, Indiana.

Gage N.L. (1994) The scientific status of the behavioral sciences: the case of research on teaching. *Teaching and Teacher Education*, **10**, 565–77.

Galton M., Simon B. & Croll P. (1980) *Inside the Primary Classroom*. Routledge and Kegan Paul, London.

Glass G.V. (1994) Review of Chambers, John H. 1992 Empiricist research on teaching. *Journal of Educational Thought*, **28**, 127–30.

Grahame-Smith D. (1995) Evidence-based medicine: Socratic dissent. *British Medical Journal*, **310**, 1126–7.

Ham C., Hunter C.J. & Robinson R. (1995) Evidence-based policymaking. *British Medical Journal*, **310**, 71–2.

Hammersley M. (1985) From ethnography to theory. *Sociology*, **19**, 244–59.

Hammersley M. (1987a) Ethnography and cumulative development of theory: a discussion of Woods' proposal for 'phase two' research. *British Education Research Journal*, **13**, 283–96.

Hammersley M. (1987b) Ethnography for survival? A reply to Woods. *British Education Research Journal*, **13**, 309–17.

Hammersley M. (1992) *What's Wrong with Ethnography?* Routledge, London.

Hammersley M. (1993) On the teacher as researcher. In M. Hammersley (ed.) *Educational Research: Current Issues*. Paul Chapman, London.

Hammersley M. (1995) *The Politics of Social Research*. Sage, London.

Hammersley M. (1996) Educational research and teaching: a response to David Hargreaves' TTA lecture. *British Educational Research Journal*, **23**, 141–61.

Hammersley M. (1997) 'A reply to David Hargreaves', unpublished paper available from author.

Hargreaves D.H. (1978) Whatever happened to symbolic interactionism? In L. Barton & R. Meighan (eds) *Sociological Interpretations of Schooling and Classrooms*. Nafferton Books, Nafferton, Driffield.

Hargreaves D.H. (1996) Teaching as a research-based profession: possibilities and prospects. Teacher Training Agency Annual Lecture 1996.

Hargreaves D.H. (1997) In defence of research for evidence-based teaching. *British Educational Research Journal*, **23**, 405–19.

Hargreaves D.H., Hester S. & Mellor F. (1975) *Deviance in Classrooms*. Routledge and Kegan Paul, London.

Hillage J., Pearson R., Anderson A. & Tamkin P. (1998) *Excellence in Research on Schools*. Department for Education and Employment, London.

Hirst P.H. (1983) Educational theory. In P.H. Hirst (ed.) *Educational Theory and its Foundation Disciplines*. Routledge and Kegan Paul, London.

Hirst P.H. (1990) The theory–practice relationship in teacher training. In M.B. Booth, V.J. Furlong & M. Wilkin (eds) *Partnership in Initial Teacher Training*. Cassell, London.

Hodgkinson H.L. (1957) Action research: a critique. *Journal of Educational Sociology,* **31**, 137–53.

Hustler D., Cassidy A. & Cuff E.C. (eds) (1986) *Action Research in Classrooms.* Allen and Unwin, London.

Jackson P. (1968) *Life in Classrooms.* Holt, Rinehart & Winston, New York.

Jadad A.R. (1996) Are you playing evidence-based medicine games with our daughter? *British Medical Journal,* **347**, 247.

Janowitz M. (1972) *Sociological Models and Social Policy.* General Learning Systems, Morristown, NJ.

Jones G. & Sagar S. (1995) No guidance is provided for situations for which evidence is lacking. *British Medical Journal,* **311**, 258.

Lancet (1995) Editorial. *Lancet,* **346**, 785.

Millett A. (1996) *Pedagogy: the Last Corner of the Secret Garden.* Third Annual Education Lecture, King's College, London.

Nisbet J. & Broadfoot P. (1980) *The Impact of Research on Policy and Practice in Education.* Aberdeen University Press, Aberdeen.

Nixon J. (ed.) *A Teacher's Guide to Action Research.* Grant McIntyre, London.

Norman G.R. (1995) Letter. *Lancet,* **346**, 839.

Norris N. (1995) Contracts, control and evaluation. *Journal of Education Policy,* **10**, 271–85.

Olson J. (1992) *Understanding Teaching.* Open University Press, Milton Keynes.

Pettigrew M. (1994) Coming to terms with research: the contract business. In D. Halpin & B. Troyna (eds) *Researching Education Policy.* Falmer, London.

Rapoport R. (1970) Three dilemmas in action research. *Human Relations,* **23**, 499–513.

Rosenberg W. & Donald A. (1995) Evidence-based medicine: an approach to clinical problem-solving. *British Medical Journal,* **310**, 1122–6.

Sackett D.L., Haynes R.B. & Tugwell P. (1985) *Clinical Epidemiology: A Basic Science for Clinical Medicine,* 2nd edition. Little, Brown and Company, Boston.

Sammons P. & Reynolds D. (1997) A partisan evaluation: John Elliott on school effectiveness. *Cambridge Journal of Education,* **27**, 123–36.

Scarth J. & Hammersley M. (1986a) Some problems in assessing closedness of tasks. In M. Hammersley (ed.) *Case Studies in Classroom Research.* Open University Press, Milton Keynes.

Scarth J. & Hammersley M. (1986b) Questioning ORACLE's analysis of teachers' questions. *Education Research,* **28**, 174–84.

Schön D. (1983) *The Reflective Practitioner.* Temple Smith, London.

Schön D. (1987) *Educating the Reflective Practitioner.* Jossey Bass, San Francisco.

Schütz A. (1967) *The Phenomenology of the Social World.* Northwestern University Press, Evanston IL.

Schwab J.J. (1969) The practical: a language for curriculum. *School Review,* **78**, 1–24.

Shuchman M. (1996) Evidence-based medicine debated. *Lancet,* **347**, 1396.

Simon H. (1955) A behavioral model of rational choice. *Quarterly Journal of Economics,* **69**, 99–118.

Stenhouse L. (1975) *An Introduction to Curriculum Research and Development.* Heinemann, London.

Teacher Training Agency (1996) *Teaching as a Research-based Profession.* Teacher Training Agency/Central Office of Information, London.

Thornton H.M. (1992) Breast cancer trials: a patient's viewpoint. *Lancet,* **339,** 44–5.

Tooley J. with Darby D. (1998) *Educational Research: a Critique.* OFSTED, London.

Wiles K. (1953) Can we sharpen up the concept of action research? *Educational Leadership,* **10,** 408–10.

Winch P. (1958) *The Idea of a Social Science and its Relationship to Philosophy.* Routledge and Kegan Paul, London.

Woods P. (1985) Ethnography and theory construction in education research. In R.G. Burgess (ed.) *Field Methods in the Study of Education.* Falmer, Lewes.

Woods P. (1987) Ethnography at the crossroads: a reply to Hammersley. *British Education Research Journal,* **13,** 297–307.

Wragg E.C. (1976) The Lancaster Study: its implications for teacher training. *British Journal of Teacher Education,* **2,** 281–90.

Chapter 9

Evidence-Based Human Resource Management

Rob Briner

Introduction

Most of the chapters in this book are each concerned with the role of evidence-based practice in a relatively specific and well-defined area of practice, such as primary care or education, that is populated by a relatively narrow range of types of practitioners. In contrast, this chapter will take a rather broader look at several practices and professions that are involved with the management of people in organisations. This general field of practice will be referred to in this chapter as human resource management (HRM), though it is also recognised that HRM usually refers to a more specific area of expertise. There are two main reasons for this rather less discipline-specific approach.

First, as will be discussed in more detail later, no single profession or group of practitioners can reasonably claim exclusive rights over the bodies of knowledge and techniques deployed in the management of people in organisations. It would, therefore, be somewhat artificial and limited to discuss evidence-based practice in relation to only one of the many practitioner groups who operate within this domain.

Second, much of the analysis of the development, or otherwise, of evidence-based practice can be applied across these practitioner groups and so there is some value in examining them together in order to draw out common issues where they are apparent. Examining these different practitioner groups together in this way is not meant in any way to imply that they all do the same type of work or that they approach their work in the same way. The approach of an HRM practitioner, for example, is certainly very different to that, say, of a trainer or specialist in selection. However, what they do have in common is an interest in the techniques, practices and interventions surrounding the management of people in organisations.

Before describing the background to research and practice in this area, I will discuss briefly some of the techniques and practitioner groups involved in this area and the increasing importance of HRM.

The practice background

Techniques, practices and policies involved in managing people

Most of us have been subjected to or indeed have subjected others to the numerous techniques that are used with the intention of managing people's behaviour in organisations. While there is a debate to be had about the extent to which these techniques are about control rather than management and indeed whether management is about little more than control, this important debate falls somewhat outside of the scope of this chapter (but see Legge 1995, 1998; Miller 1996).

The way in which people are managed in organisations has potentially profound implications, not only in terms of organisational effectiveness and survival, but also in terms of the quality of working life and the development of individuals. Hence, the techniques that are used to manage people, if effective, have broad consequences for the well-being of both organisations and individuals, and even perhaps local communities and national economies.

These techniques, practices, and policies are now widely deployed in many public, private and voluntary sector organisations. Box 9.1 shows some of those that are more commonly used. These have been somewhat crudely divided here into those that intervene at the individual or group level, and those that intervene at the organisational level.

Box 9.1: Some practices and interventions used to manage people in organisations

Individual/group level	*Organisational level*
Job analysis	Organisational development
Recruitment	Restructuring
Selection interviews	Delayering
Structured application forms	Change management
Personality tests	Communications strategies
Assessment centres	Succession planning
Ability tests	Culture change
Training and development	Mission statements
Performance appraisal	Renegotiating the psychological contract
Goal-setting	Early retirement schemes
360 degree feedback	Pay and reward systems
Job redesign	Quality management
Promotion and regrading	Management by objectives
Career-planning	Organisational design
Team-building	Equal opportunity or diversity policies
Counselling	Employee involvement

A very wide range of techniques is apparent. Some focus on job appli-
cants' aptitudes and abilities with the aim of selecting people with the
apparently best match to the particular requirements of the job or role.
Others attempt to train or develop employees. A number of these techniques, such as performance appraisal and goal-setting, aim to manage
motivation and performance in a relatively direct way. In contrast, the
impact of organisational-level techniques such as culture change and
restructuring on employee behaviour are far less direct and any resulting
effects are likely to be observed in the longer term.

While all these techniques share the aim of managing people, their
theoretical roots can be traced back to a range of disciplines and sources.
The most obvious basis for individual- and group-level interventions is
psychology and, in particular, occupational or organisational psychology
and social psychology. (Of these, occupational psychology is a peculiarly
British term – in the rest of Europe the same field would be described as
work and organisational psychology and in the US industrial and organisational psychology.) Other practices have their origins in the discipline of
ergonomics, or human factors, which is concerned with designing the
physical and psychological demands of tasks, jobs and environments so
that they can be met both safely and effectively. The roots of organisational-
level interventions are also diverse and can be found in organisational
sociology, organisational behaviour (though this is also related to individual and group practices), organisation studies, industrial relations,
management studies, and the work of so-called management gurus (see
below, this chapter under *Fad and fashion*).

The techniques deployed in HRM are therefore many and varied.
However, this is hardly surprising given that any technique or intervention
which can be claimed to affect, or indeed does affect, people's behaviour in
organisations can be considered to be part of HRM. This diversity is also
found in the many practitioner groups involved in managing people in
organisations that will be discussed in the next section.

It is certainly worth asking briefly here at the outset the extent to which
the practices listed in Box 9.1 have an evidence base: that is, the extent to
which each can draw on a reliable body of evidence concerning their
effectiveness? While, in general, most of these practices cannot claim to
have even a modest evidence base, for others (some of which will be discussed in more detail later) the evidence base is much more developed.
Those practices aimed at an individual or group level listed in the left-hand
side of Box 9.1 tend to have a more developed evidence base largely,
perhaps, because they are simply more researchable. Organisational-level
interventions are, on the whole, much more difficult and costly to investigate and have more diffuse goals.

A discussion of the evidence base for each of the practices listed in Box
9.1 would consist of a summary of the entire field of HRM research and

related areas, which clearly is not possible here. However, examples of specific practices will be discussed here to provide a sense of the types of evidence which do and do not exist. These examples are not comprehensive reviews of available evidence but rather give a flavour of the available evidence base.

Examples of the nature of the existing evidence base for individual and group practices

Here, three examples will be considered: job redesign, team-building, and performance management. The aims of job redesign are often many and varied. Typically, however, the twin aims are to 'improve' jobs for both the organisation and individual. For the organisation, the focus may include efficiency, quality, employee absence rates, and so on. For the employee, issues such as job satisfaction and well-being are likely to be important. A particularly important aim of job redesign has been to increase the autonomy or control employees have over their job tasks and most studies look at the impact of this type of job redesign intervention.

So does job redesign work? There are perhaps a dozen studies which are well designed enough to allow us to draw some tentative conclusions. In a review of this literature, Briner and Reynolds (1999) reached the conclusion reached by many others in the field: that if variables assessing efficiency, absence, satisfaction, and so on are measured before and at several points following the job redesign intervention, some things appear to get worse, some better, and most things appear not to change. There is also some evidence that the same kind of job redesign intervention will not have the same effects if introduced in different sites of the same organisation or in different organisations. One limitation of these interventions is that often they were introduced without initial assessment and hence they were not necessarily aimed at resolving any particular problem.

Given the apparently increasing emphasis given to teams as a way of organising work, it is not surprising that the second example, team-building, appears to be a popular intervention. Team-building focuses on the processes that occur within groups with the aim of improving team effectiveness. Different approaches can be taken. For example, some interventions may focus on conflict resolution, others on roles and responsibilities. Somewhat limited evidence is available about the effectiveness of team-building interventions (see Tannenbaum *et al.* 1996). This suggests that no one method necessarily works better than any other and such interventions can have a positive impact on individual perceptions and attitudes towards the team. In other words, people may view their team and their role within it more positively following such an intervention. However, it is not clear that these interventions actually change the behaviour of teams and team members and hence their impact on team effectiveness may be minimal. The team-building interventions studied suffer from a similar weakness to those interventions studied in job re-design. It was also not clear that the teams subjected to these interventions had a 'problem' in the first place.

Performance management is something of an umbrella term which in part refers to any technique which aims to manage the performance of employees and in part refers to the notion using a range of techniques in a systematic or integrative way for managing performance. Such techniques would certainly include some of those listed in Box 9.1, such as perfor-mance appraisal, goal-setting, and 360° feedback. Yet again, the aims are often broad and complex, but are focused on improving individual and organisational performance – though defining and assessing performance is, of course, by no means a simple task. Does performance management work? In a review of the field of performance management, Williams (1998) concludes that we do not know as we simply do not have sufficient evi-dence to draw any kind of conclusion.

It seems likely that, with the possible exception of some selection tech-niques, the same sort of patterns would emerge if we considered the available evidence for any of the individual/group-level practices listed in Box 9.1. In many cases there would just be very little or no systematic evidence about the effectiveness of the technique and even where evidence does exist it would provide very mixed support for its effectiveness.

Examples of the nature of the existing evidence base for organisational-level practices

Some of the difficulties in assessing the effectiveness of group and individual-level techniques become even more apparent when we try to examine the impact of organisational-level changes on individuals and organisations. We will briefly consider two organisational-level practices: organisational development and management by objectives.

Organisational development has been defined by Porras and Robertson as:

> 'a set of behavioural science-based theories, values, strategies, and techniques aimed at the planned change of the organisational work setting for the purpose of enhancing individual development and improving organisational performance, through the alteration of organisational members' on the job behaviours'.
>
> (Porras & Robertson 1992: 722)

Organisational development is, like performance management, something of an umbrella term and one which comes very close indeed to the broad definition of HRM offered at the start of this chapter. Many of the tech-niques listed in the right-hand column of Box 9.1 (and some of those in the left-hand column) can therefore be considered to be organisational development of one form or another. Porras and Robertson (1992) reviewed ten years' worth of studies (which met certain criteria) and found that, on average, organisational development interventions resulted in positive changes in the outcome variables measured less than 40% of the time. Does organisational development work? Again, the evidence is not clear but suggests that sometimes it does, but often it does not.

A second example, management by objectives, consists of a combination of goal-setting, participation in decision-making, and objective feedback. Management by objectives therefore consists of individual-, group- and organisational-level components (reinforcing the point made earlier that the distinction between the levels of intervention described in Box 9.1 is not necessarily a particularly valid one). A meta-analysis revealed that in 68 of the 70 studies included productivity gains were found (Rogers & Hunter 1991). The meta-analysis also revealed that when top management commitment to management by objectives was high the productivity gain was, on average, 56% but when low it was only 6%.

As we go on to discuss in more detail later, the impacts of organisational-level interventions are more difficult to study than individual- or group-level interventions. However, we can again conclude in the case of these interventions that evidence is somewhat limited and not wholly supportive.

Levels of analysis and single versus multiple practice issues in researching HRM practices

The kind of research which is often conducted into individual and group practices tends to focus more on their impacts on individual employees rather than their longer term impact on, say, organisational performance and profits. It is implicitly assumed, however, that changes on the individual or group level will eventually have an impact on organisational-level indicators of performance. Such an assumption is highly questionable due to the large number of intervening variables and processes that occur between the individual, the group, and then the organisational performance (see Johns 1997). A key issue in HRM research is, therefore, the level of analysis on which we expect to observe effects.

A second important issue concerns the extent to which single practices looked at in isolation are relevant. There are strong arguments and some evidence for the idea that single HRM techniques are relatively unimportant. What matters is the particular combination of techniques which is used (e.g. Huselid 1995). While it is desirable that each technique is effective in its own terms is it, in practice, relevant given that a number of practices will always be operating together? Another, and perhaps more important test of such practices has to take place through an examination of how they collectively, and in specific combinations, effect a broad range of outcomes. Both of these issues will be discussed later in more detail.

Practitioner groups involved in HRM and how they operate

Some of the key practitioners in this field are generalists who deal with a range of issues that concern HRM. In the UK, occupational or organisational psychologists, for example, when chartered are expected to be able to work across eight key areas that have been specified by the British Psychological Society (BPS). Likewise, members of the Institute of Personnel and Development are expected to have skills in a number of areas (see Box 9.2).

Box 9.2: Examples of some of the areas in which professional bodies expect their members to have expertise

British Psychological Society Occupational Psychology Division	*Institute of Personnel and Development*
Personnel selection and assessment	Selection and assessment centres
Training	Human resource planning
Human–machine interaction	Organisational consultancy
Design of working environments and work, including health and safety	Health and safety
	Employee development
Counselling	Management development
Personal development	Managing learning process
Performance appraisal	Employee reward
Career development	Performance management
Employee relations	Employment relations
Motivation	Employment law
Organisational development and change	Employee counselling and welfare
Organisational consultancy	Managing change

As with most professional bodies, members of the Division of Occupational Psychology and those who belong to various levels of membership of the Institute of Personnel and Development must be able to demonstrate clearly their experience and competence in specific areas.

In addition to these relative generalists who may also undertake specialist work, there are many who specialise in particular fields and in the use of particular techniques or the introduction of particular interventions. They may or may not belong to professional bodies such as the IPD or BPS but it would appear that, in many or most cases, such an affiliation is certainly not necessary in order to practice under one of the labels listed in Box 9.3.

The ways in which practitioners are organised and work within HRM has vital implications for evidence-based practice in this field. The most relevant features of their work will be described and their implications briefly outlined. These implications will be more fully considered in later sections.

Box 9.3: Practitioners involved in HRM

Generic human resource managers/practitioners
Management consultants
Organisational psychologists
Training specialists
Recruitment and selection practitioners
Pay and remuneration specialists
Psychological assessment specialists
Change management consultants
Organisational development consultants
Career counsellors
Ergonomists/human factor specialists
Organisational communication consultants

First, although professional bodies do exist in the industry, freelance practitioners in particular remain largely unregulated. Any person may claim to be an expert in training or change management, for example, and be employed by an organisation to undertake this work. The credibility of the practitioner with a client may depend more on word of mouth and claims they make about previous clients and success rates than membership of professional bodies and educational or professional qualifications. Marketing literature listing blue-chip client companies and containing triumphant descriptions of achievements with previous clients is a standard way of claiming legitimacy for many practitioners in this field.

For many other areas of professional activity thus far discussed in other chapters, membership of professional bodies and specific qualifications are required in order to practice. At the present time, therefore, practitioners within HRM can obtain work on the basis of somewhat limited evidence about the effectiveness of their practices and much of what is practised appears to be outside the jurisdiction of professional bodies.

A second important feature of the work of practitioners in this field is that while larger organisations employ in-house HRM specialists who are likely, as a job requirement, to belong to professional bodies, many smaller organisations may have no internal expertise and rely exclusively on buying in the services they require. Even large organisations may only have a core of HRM specialists and outsource many HRM functions, such as training or recruitment, to outside firms. What this then means is that unlike the other fields thus far discussed, there are very many freelance practitioners, small consultancies, and loose collections of associates. Many practitioners (though no figures are available) therefore rely for their income on obtaining a succession of perhaps relatively small contracts. One implication of this is that such practitioners must market and sell as well as deliver their services, which may cause some conflict of interests. A further implication of the large number of small or single-person practitioner companies is that systematic attempts to gather evaluation data on the use of particular techniques would present a complex if not impossible task.

Third, much of the work in this field probably takes place outside the public sector or at least is less well developed in a formal sense in the public sector. One implication of this is that issues of accountability are somewhat different from other areas of practice. A further issue is that training in HRM is not organised by the state in the same way. Although postgraduate degrees provide the academic base for work as an occupational or organisational psychologist, for example, they are not, like teaching or medical education, designed to produce practitioners in the same sense.

There is, therefore, a range of practitioners working in HRM in a number of different ways. The context in which they operate and the organisation of work in the field has a number of important implications for evidence-based practice. Another important feature of HRM, which will be discussed next, is its relatively recent expansion and development.

The rise and rise of HRM

The contemporary management mantra 'our people are our greatest asset' is one which is often greeted with a great deal of scepticism and cynicism. For any particular organisation, this claim may or may not be true in financial or strategic terms and the motives behind such a declaration may be more or less questionable. However, what is undoubtedly true is that such talk, whether empty or not, signals that organisations and their managers are now, probably more than ever before, expressing an enthusiasm for making the management of people a serious and central task of management. There are a number of reasons for this but perhaps the most significant is the attempt by managers and others to understand what distinguishes successful, effective organisations as well as economies from others. A common answer to the question of why one particular organisation is more successful than others in its field is 'the people'. Successful organisations appear to be populated by workers who are more motivated, more skilled, show greater commitment, are 'empowered' and demonstrate a willingness to 'go that extra mile'.

Some evidence for this shift can be found in the change from using the term 'personnel management' to the term 'human resource management' to describe the activities of those sections of management responsible for managing people. While managers may assume that others should view being referred to as assets or resources as a mark of management's respect, it does not always seem to be the case that those thus dubbed view such a label as flattering. However, the use of this economic terminology to describe workers is not so much to impress employees but rather to persuade senior managers and members of boards that spending money on managing people is something worth doing as it will enhance effectiveness and profitability. By referring to employees as resources or assets the intention, presumably, is to make clear that managing human resources is just as important as managing any other organisational resource.

Another shift is that HRM, unlike personnel management, is regarded as being part of the broader organisational strategy. Personnel management was to some extent regarded as dealing largely with the administrative matters surrounding employment such as holiday entitlement, monitoring of absence, arranging selection interviews, and organising retirement. It was also perhaps regarded as 'soft' in that it dealt with the personal and welfare needs of employees. In contrast, HRM places less emphasis on these soft aspects of managing people and more on 'harder', results-oriented issues such as performance management, increasing workforce flexibility and ultimately the links between HRM strategy and financial and other kinds of performance. It is important to note that the meaning of HRM is far from precise and indeed debates as to its nature (e.g. Legge 1995) and the extent to which it is indeed hard or soft (e.g. Truss *et al.* 1997) form one important area of HRM research.

Given the assumed and/or desired links between HRM and organisational performance and the hardening of the approach to managing people it would appear that evidence-based practice would find a natural home in HRM. Shareholders and senior managers will expect there to be good evidence for the effectiveness of the HRM policies and practices in which they invest. However, as I will go on to discuss, there are numerous reasons why this has not yet happened, and perhaps may never happen.

The research background

Despite vigorous practical activity it would be difficult to characterise HRM as a field which has a very strong research culture. Here I consider the role of research in HRM, some of the ways in which practitioners make decisions, and evidence for the presence of evidence-based practice in HRM.

The role of research in HRM

Scientific management and the oppression of workers

For employees, managers and trades' unions the term 'science' may have unfortunate connotations in relation to managing people. The work of Frederick Taylor (1856–1915) had a scientific approach to management which involved, to put it simply, finding out 'scientifically' the most efficient way to perform a particular job and then ensuring that workers performed the job in that manner (e.g. Rose 1988). The idea of doing research about how to manage people is somehow unavoidably bound up with the time-and-motion study in which each and every move made by workers undertaking particular tasks was measured and monitored in order to improve the design of the task and job.

Managing people in organisations does, to varying degrees, involve control, manipulation (in both neutral and negative senses), and can also be considered in a more political and economic sense to involve exploitation and oppression. Even the rhetoric and reality of empowerment, for example, can be simply viewed as a slightly more sophisticated means of exploitation. Although the other practitioners discussed in this book can also be thought of as engaging in control and manipulation in their practice, a fundamental difference, in the eyes of most clients, is the assumption that practitioners such as nurses, doctors and teachers at least mean well and are fundamentally oriented towards helping other people. The work of the HRM practitioner is less likely to be regarded in such a broadly positive way (as with some contemporary attitudes towards social workers). At this point it is worth considering the place of research in HRM, as the role of research in what may be seen as a broadly positive area of practice is somewhat different to its role in an area in which questions are raised about the motives behind and outcomes of practice. If a practice is regarded with suspicion then so too will be efforts to make it more effective.

Of course, much of what HRM practitioners do can be regarded as benevolent, or at least benign. For example, activities such as providing training to enable people to do their jobs more effectively; ensuring fairness in selection procedures; trying to maximise the fit between a person's abilities and potential and the demands of the job; and making sure systems are in place to provide adequate feedback to employees, would not, in themselves, be perceived by many employees as exploitative. On the other hand, helping make decisions about who is made redundant during a period of job-cutting; being to some extent responsible where cases of discrimination or bias do occur; or introducing reward systems which are felt to be unfair, are all activities which may be viewed as somewhat less than benevolent.

HRM practice can therefore be viewed as inherently ambiguous and evidence or research around it is also likely to take on some of this ambiguity. This theme will be revisited later when I consider some likely responses to evidence-based practice in HRM. It is also worth noting that this ambiguity is evident more broadly when thinking about management generally, where in different historical periods varying emphases are given to different ideological views of the place of employees (e.g. Barley & Kunda 1992).

HRM research

The question, Does it work? is frequently asked of particular HRM practices and of HRM as a whole. In terms of the whole range of HRM practices, that is any practice or intervention that is in some way involved with managing people in organisations, there is, as suggested above, relatively little very strong or comprehensive evidence about their effectiveness. Mabey *et al.* (1998) ask a slightly different question: Is HRM delivering on its promises? They answer thus: 'we have to conclude, on the evidence of this volume, that many of its prized goals (more satisfied customers, more empowered workers, more trusting employment relationships, more unified culture, greater workforce creativity and commitment) remain unproven at best, and unfulfilled at worst' (Mabey *et al.* 1998: 237).

At least two main types of research can, however, be identified: one which considers the effectiveness of specific techniques, the other which considers the extent to which HRM practices collectively result in, for example, increased performance and commitment. Each of these will be discussed in turn. There is also an important third type of research which explores the ambiguities in and meanings of HRM as mentioned earlier and takes a critical approach to interpreting the use of HRM in organisations (e.g. Legge 1995, 1998). Though important, this work falls outside the scope of this chapter.

Probably the most heavily researched area or set of practices within HRM, and within organisational psychology in particular, is selection and assessment. There are numerous reasons for this, but perhaps the two most important are the emphasis given by organisations to finding the 'right' people (and avoiding the 'wrong' people); and the relative ease with which research can be conducted. One very long-running issue, for example, concerns the extent to which a variety of predictors such as biodata, personality measures, ability measures, and so on, do actually predict subsequent job performance (see Borman *et al.* 1997). This may involve specific HRM inputs such as assessment centres, personality and ability tests, and structured application forms. Organisations often collect such data during the selection process and some sort of performance measures may also be regularly collected from employees. Hence, this represents a relatively tidy framework in which to ask some quite straightforward questions although in practice, of course, it is somewhat more complex. As suggested earlier, the extent to which these measures, and in particular personality measures, can predict subsequent performance and their utility (or results of cost–benefit analysis) has been subject to considerable research and debate (e.g. Barrick & Mount 1991; Tett *et al.* 1991). Many of the results suggest quite modest but consistent relationships between personality measures and subsequent performance.

Rather than try to quantify the general relationship between personality and performance there has also been a growing interest in attempting to clarify the nature of the numerous predictors used in selection (e.g. test results, ratings from interviews, qualifications); and the many and varied criteria which can be used as indicators of performance (e.g. technical proficiency, job advancement, ratings from co-workers). This is in order to identify the specific linkages between different kinds of predictors and different kinds of indicators of performance. Such work, it is argued, 'continues to help us raise personnel selection from a technology to a science' (Borman *et al.* 1997: 330). It is worth noting that much activity within HRM is more broadly concerned with technology than science.

Another important area is training – though it is certainly less researched than selection and assessment. This research does not simply take the form of asking whether or not particular kinds of training – such as assertiveness, time management, or technology – actually work but, rather, asks questions about under what circumstances particular kinds of training are likely to work and why training works (e.g. Noe & Ford 1992). For example, when is instructional versus experiential, or formal versus informal, more or less likely to be effective?

Researchers into training exhort practitioners to become researchers and evaluators by first clearly establishing what the specific training needs are, the specific outcomes the training is supposed to achieve, designing the training so it is likely to achieve the desired result, and then evaluating the training against the outcomes which have been set. There is some evidence that only a very small minority of organisations do this (e.g. Tannenbaum & Yukl 1992). More instead tend to implement a training programme with little initial analysis, and judge its effectiveness by trainee reactions to the training (i.e. whether they found it useful or liked it), rather than whether or not it has impacted on behaviour.

One key issue in relation to training is that of transfer, that is the extent to which the behaviours and skills, if developed in training, actually transfer to behaviour in the workplace. Although it is widely recognised that what happens in the work environment after the trainee returns to work is likely to determine the extent to which transfer takes place, little is known about what particular characteristics are likely to be important (Tannenbaum & Yukl 1992).

A crude summary of much of the research into specific HRM techniques would be that there is, on the whole, little good evidence; and that which exists suggests that some of these techniques may work, to some extent. A general shift, however, in those areas where there is some systematic research has been away from simply asking, Does it work? to asking, Why does it work? or, Under what circumstances does it work?

As stated earlier, a more accurate definition of HRM would be that it is a strategic approach to managing people in line with the wider goals of the organisation and external contingencies, and that it is through the strategic use of particular combinations of the specific techniques already discussed which will determine the overall effectiveness of HRM. This latter type of research, which is largely unconcerned about the effectiveness of particular techniques, certainly dominates HRM research within the management literature. For example, if a strategic decision is taken that the organisation will become more customer-focused then this has implications for a whole range of HRM activities including selection, training, supervision, performance assessment, job design, reward systems, and communications. Hence, in addition to asking questions about the effectiveness of any particular technique, we can also ask whether HRM as a general coordinated activity in this sense works.

Guest (1997) identifies three types of theory about HRM which we need to consider in order to more fully discuss the kinds of questions addressed by HRM research and, in particular, questions surrounding HRM effectiveness. The first of these comprises strategic theories that examine the extent to which HRM practices and policy are shaped by internal and external contexts. As with all contingency or 'fit' theories, the assumption is that the better the fit between HRM and the context the better the level of organisational performance. Guest (1997) suggests that these theoretical approaches are simply too under-specified as they do not explain how and why HRM has possible links to performance.

The second type of theory is descriptive and attempts to provide a conceptual framework for HRM policies and practices and related outcomes. While such an approach provides classifications of HRM it does not, again, suggest how HRM is linked to performance.

The third theoretical approach is described as normative as it attempts to state, on the basis of evidence or values, which combination of specific HRM practices are likely to lead to superior organisational performance in any context. These theories do attempt to state how and why HRM may lead to performance. Most of these theories imply that the aims of HRM are to deploy particular kinds of HRM practice in order to develop high levels of commitment, quality and flexibility from the workforce leading in turn to superior organisational performance (see Fig. 9.1).

A fundamental issue in considering the effectiveness or otherwise of HRM is which criteria we use to gauge whether HRM works. At one level we can examine the feelings and attitudes – such as stress, satisfaction, attitudes to management, intention to quit, and so on – of individual employees. Such soft measures, while important, are perhaps of less interest than harder organisational indicators of performance. Locke and Latham (1990) describe three categories of such harder performance data: measures of output (quantitative, qualitative); measures of time (e.g. lost working time, absence, meeting deadlines); and financial indicators (e.g. return on investment, profit).

So does HRM work, in the sense that it has a positive impact on such

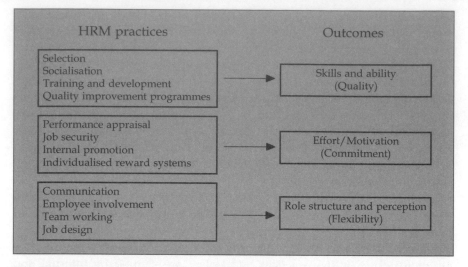

Fig. 9.1 Possible links between specific HRM practices and outcomes (adapted from Guest, 1997)

performance indicators? Guest (1997) suggests that there are three main empirical approaches to examining links between HRM and performance each of which considers the extent to which different kinds of fit between HRM and other factors leads to enhanced performance. The first of these types of fit, external fit, is where HRM strategy is made to fit the broader organisational strategy, which in turn is based on responses to the external context of the organisation. For example, an organisation may decide, on the basis of considering other competitors in its sector, to adopt a strategy leading to high-quality products and services. According to the external fit approach, HRM policies should therefore be those which also lead to higher quality. There is some evidence for the benefits of this approach though it is not unequivocal.

A second type of fit is internal fit, where fit is considered to be the extent to which internal HRM policies and practices fit with an ideal set of practices. Guest (1997) suggests that there is more evidence for this type of fit than any other. Studies indicate that the more high-performance HRM practices adopted (see back to those indicated in Fig. 9.1) the greater the performance as indicated by a range of measures.

The third type of fit, configurational fit, suggests that it may be particular patterns, combinations, bundles, or clusters of practices that fit with each other in particular ways to improve performance. An assumption here is that there is no ideal type and that different practices in different combinations may have the same or similar effects. Supportive evidence for this is mixed and not particularly strong.

Guest (1997) observes that much of the evidence in this field is cross-sectional (so even where relationships between HRM and performance may be found, causality cannot be established), the measurement of HRM and performance varies widely across studies, and some are sector-specific while others are not. While evidence does exist, the conclusions that can be drawn from it are somewhat limited and should be treated with caution.

From this brief overview of HRM research, what conclusions relevant to evidence-based practice can be drawn? First, while there are data around about specific and combinations of practices, it is of variable quality and unevenly spread across different practices, organisational types, and sectors. As a consequence there are some specific difficulties in this context in trying to make the existing body of knowledge cumulative (Becker & Gerhart 1996; see also other papers in the special edition of *Academy of Management Journal* on HRM and organisational performance). Second, what we mean by effectiveness in relation to HRM is not straightforward. As indicated above, a large number of measures, at different levels of analysis, can be taken as indicators of individual and organisational effectiveness or performance. Third, conducting research into HRM is difficult and expensive for a variety of reasons. While studies of single practices in one organisation are relatively manageable (though perhaps of limited value), those which attempt to address bigger questions of whether or not HRM has an impact on organisational performance are, to say the least, daunting. Such studies need to be longitudinal, perhaps over many years, as the impact of HRM may take some years to show. Large numbers of organisations are required. Valid and reliable measures of HRM practices and organisational performance need to be collected at many time points. The numerous other variables which may impact upon organisational performance and intervene in the HRM performance relationship, and which therefore need to be controlled for in any analysis, also need to be measured. It also helps, though is unlikely to be the case, if the organisations in the study remain relatively stable in terms of size and ownership and are relatively consistent in their HRM practices.

As I will discuss later, the present and likely future nature of the evidence and theory about HRM appears to play a key role in shaping responses to evidence-based practice and also its significance and development within HRM.

Practitioner training and involvement in research

Within HRM, like many other areas, there does not always seem to be much of an overlap between the questions and themes that concern practitioners and those which concern researchers. This lack of common purpose is often the topic of debates where ways in which the practitioner–academic divide can be bridged are discussed. Such debates can be somewhat tedious as they contain over-rehearsed and limited arguments and appear to miss a fundamental issue: academics and practitioners are engaged in different work which has different goals and different reward systems which is reflected, of course, in the different and sometimes conflicting priorities of the two groups.

Such debates do, however, also reveal areas of common interest. One theme that does concern both practitioners and academics is the extent to which and in what circumstances single or combined HRM practices are likely to impact on a range of outcomes such as employee attitudes and behaviours through to financial performance.

In spite of these concerns, for the vast majority of HRM practitioners research training is not part of their broader training nor does it feature as part of continuing professional development. Not only is there an absence of research training in terms of conducting research, but there also appears to be no training in how to go about systematically and critically evaluating evidence which is either internal to the organisation or found externally in published research.

There are a few exceptions to this general absence of research training. Occupational psychologists receive research training at both undergraduate and postgraduate levels, while those who receive specialist training in assessment or training methods will also be taught some of the skills required for evaluation. However, even in these cases, it is not uncommon to be told by practitioners that the language and structure of most academic journal articles renders them impenetrable, incomprehensible, and therefore unusable.

While individual practitioners are unlikely to be involved in research, the Institute of Personnel and Development funds some research and commissions reviews of research in specific areas of interest to its members, such as diversity and training, and research into the relationship between HRM and financial performance.

How do HRM practitioners make decisions about practices and interventions?

There is limited evidence about how practitioners make decisions. However, from personal observation and both formal and informal discussion some themes can be identified. I also draw on some of the literature on managerial behaviour and decision-making which seems to apply equally well to the kinds of decisions faced by HRM practitioners – many of whom are also managers.

Given the absence of training it is not surprising that practitioners do not seem to make great use of published research in reaching decisions about their work. Here, several different ways in which HRM practitioners may make decisions are considered. However, inherent in many of these different ways of making decisions, as in much decision-making, are issues of power, control, reputation-enhancement and protection, and the identities of the decision-maker.

Fad and fashion

So prevalent are fad and fashion in the area of HRM, and management practice more generally, that they are even routinely ridiculed, for example, in the highly successful work of syndicated comic strip author Scott Adams (*The Dilbert Principle: a cubicle's-eye view of bosses, meetings, management fads, and other workplace afflictions*, Adams 1997). They have also become a popular or indeed faddish area of study in their own right (e.g. Abrahamson 1996; Aldag 1997; Gill & Whittle 1993). The kinds of questions addressed within this field of research include why fads and fashions come and go, how practitioners learn about fads and fashions, and how they are justified and understood.

This interest has now come full circle and some popular management books now warn managers about the dangers of fads. Books such as *Fad Surfing in the Boardroom: Reclaiming the Courage to Manage in the Age of Instant Answers* (Shapiro 1995) and *Back to Basics: A Fad-Free Diet for Corporate Managers* (Himmelfarb 1997) warn managers and practitioners of the dangers of the quick fix.

The origins of this research arise from a puzzling observation, namely that the solutions managers adopt to meet the often similar or identical problems they face appear to be so numerous, diverse, and change so rapidly. Such turbulence is found in general management (e.g. downsizing, excellence, total quality management, business process re-engineering, knowledge management, the learning organisation) and HRM (e.g. assessment centres, 360° appraisal, family-friendly policies, teamwork and empowerment).

A number of reasons can be identified for the appearance of fad and fashion in HRM. One of these is the influence of the management guru, now considered so strong an influence on the behaviour of some organisations and managers, that it too has become an area of study (Clark & Salaman 1998; Huczynski 1993). Management gurus typically are charismatic, dramatic performers, and present compelling reasons why their suggestions need to be adopted as a matter of urgency if organisational ruin is to be avoided. Their ideas are often simple (but not *too* simple) and promise to bring some sort of order into what managers may feel are chaotic and unpredictable organisations.

A second reason for the dominance of fad and fashion is that of mimicry. In any decision-making context we may observe others, perhaps those perceived as more successful or more like the ideal of ourselves, in order to pick up tips or clues about what to do to be more like them. In the case of organisations, mimetic isomorphism, where organisations change to be more like others, has been considered to be a significant driver of the direction of change. This combination of 'keeping up with the Joneses' and 'if X blue chip company are doing it then surely so should we' seems to be very powerful in the case of HRM practice.

A third explanation for fad and fashion can be found by examining the characteristics of those who champion the particular management or HRM practice that is then introduced. This has been referred to as issue-selling (e.g. Dutton & Ashford 1993; Dutton *et al.* 1997) where, for a range of often personal reasons, an ambitious manager will attempt to persuade others that they have correctly identified the problem for which they also have the perfect solution. For these three reasons, and others, it appears that the kinds of decisions HRM practitioners make are subject to some extent, like in any other area of management, to fad and fashion.

Availability of off-the-shelf products and services

One important factor that seems to influence choice is simply availability. The decision to intervene may be driven more by pragmatism and urgency than a longer-term consideration of effectiveness and so be strongly shaped by the relative availability of services and products. In the case of psychometric tests, for example, the major publishers of these tests go to great lengths not only to ensure their ready availability but to encourage practitioners to use their products exclusively. Likewise, a predesigned training programme may appeal more than one that has to be designed for the organisation based on an initial thorough training needs analysis.

Difficulty of accessing relevant information

While one major function of HRM is to keep good records of important employee behaviours such as absence, turnover, performance ratings, and so on, it does, somewhat surprisingly, often appear to be the case that these data are not readily accessible or, where they are, are not in a form which can easily be used to inform decision-making.

Not only is internal information limited, external information about the efficacy of various interventions is also not readily available. As will be discussed later, there are very few ways of obtaining systematic evidence, such as reviews of HRM evaluations.

A minor though perhaps illustrative example of these apparent difficulties can be found in the regular enquiries I receive from organisations who believe, first, they have an absence problem and, second that its cause is stress. When asked what current and past absence rates in the organisation actually are, most readily admit that figures are not available and even where they are, they are likely to be inaccurate. (The difficulty of collecting good absence figures and maintaining accurate records should not, however, be underestimated.) Even where, in a minority of cases, good absence data are available it usually seems to be the case that no attempt to compare these absence figures to national, local or sector averages has been made. Hence, the rate of absence may frequently be unknown and, even where it is known, the extent to which it is high or otherwise has not been established. Even where absence is relatively high, it is unlikely, according to the best available evidence (e.g. Johns 1997; Harrison & Martoccho 1998), that stress is a major or particularly significant cause of raised absence levels, though stress is currently widely claimed to be a cause of many organisational and individual ills.

It appears, therefore, to be the case that decisions are not made on the basis of sound internal or external information about the nature and extent of the problem nor its possible causes, nor the probable efficacy of interventions.

Multiple, incompatible, and opaque goals of intervention

Except in the simplest of cases, HRM interventions are likely to have complex, contradictory and often unclear goals. The goals of a single intervention or a particular package of HRM measures may include increases in commitment, performance, job satisfaction and reductions in absence and turnover, for example. Hence, the decision about what interventions and practices to adopt is almost bound to be somewhat unstructured and, as a result, influenced by many kinds of fads and fashions, as discussed earlier, and decision-making heuristics (e.g. it seemed to work before, or is the least unpalatable decision), and satisficing – i.e. finding a 'good-enough' apparent solution.

The HRM problems identified, and hence the goals of intervention, will rarely be single and specific, and incorporate many of the various problems or difficulties observed by practitioners or reported by employees. However, the ill-defined nature of problems in complex organisations cannot be overstated. It is likely that practitioners would argue that HRM problems or issues rarely present themselves as neat and tidy puzzles that lend themselves to neat solutions.

Evidence for evidence-based practice in HRM

While, as discussed earlier, there is some research which attempts to evaluate HRM and make it accountable and impact on the bottom line, it has not been possible to find examples of the explicit adoption of evidence-based practice frameworks within HRM. Perhaps the only exception is a government document produced by the UK Department of Health (Department of Health 1998) which also funds research into HRM. This document sets out a strategy for an approach to HRM within the UK National Health Service. Although the term evidence-based practice does not appear in this document, there is a great emphasis on building an evidence base for the effectiveness of HRM practices, as well as the continuous monitoring of the effectiveness of practices which are subsequently introduced. It is interesting to note that this approach has appeared first in the public sector which tends to have slightly less formally developed HRM practices, and in a medical setting, which is also the true origin of evidence-based practice.

We do not, however, have good evidence about the adoption of evidence-based practice in HRM. It is not clear that at the level of individual practices or indeed at the level of strategic HRM, practitioners and organisations are necessarily seeking out the best available evidence in making decisions about what practices and policies to adopt.

Where evidence is used it is likely to be somewhat distant from its source and may have been communicated to practitioners and organisations through, for example, consultants, textbooks, professional magazines and journals, and observations of the practices of other organisations.

The future for evidence-based practice in HRM?

There are some good reasons to assume that evidence-based practice will not emerge more strongly in HRM and some good reasons to assume that it will. Some of the reasons why evidence-based practice may not emerge more strongly can be found, in part, by considering the analysis presented earlier of how practitioners in this field presently make decisions. In effect, it appears that very little evidence is used and hence a considerable shift in thinking and behaviour would be required in order to adopt evidence-based practice. Another reason why evidence-based practice may not emerge is in relation to the quantity and quality of available evidence. While it is difficult to make a thorough analysis of this potential problem, as it would require an overview of all HRM-related research, it is certainly possible that for some kinds of interventions and practices (particularly those based on fad and fashion) very little evidence will be available.

Evidence-based practice may emerge, though, as a consequence of the need to make HRM accountable – not only in terms of its contribution to organisational effectiveness and profitability, but also through its accountability to the employees who are subjected to HRM techniques. It is quite possible that a career development intervention, for example, in which an employee is asked to discuss quite personal feelings and ambitions, may have quite negative effects. Without evidence of the effectiveness and safety of such interventions, HRM practitioners may become liable for any resulting longer-term harm that could result (see Box 9.4).

Box 9.4: A summary of some possible reasons for the emergence and non-emergence of evidence-based practice in HRM

Reasons for evidence-based practice in HRM	*Reasons against evidence-based practice in HRM*
Accountability of HRM	Limitations of existing evidence
Drive to improve effectiveness	Difficulty and costs of research
Emerging assertiveness of HRM	Generalisability of findings
Current lack of access to available evidence	Current decision-making practices
Increasing professionalism	Practitioner reactions
Competition for organisational resources	
Value for money	

Evidence-based practice may emerge more strongly in HRM but perhaps not in its purest or fullest form. Some of the reasons for this will be discussed below.

Some likely responses to evidence-based practice

If evidence-based practice were to emerge more strongly in HRM, what kinds of responses would we expect? A few, possibly a minority, would be enthusiasts and champions for evidence-based practice as appears to have happened in other areas of practice. Some would probably be offended at the implication that practice was not already evidence-based. Those who are somewhat sceptical about the benefits of HRM would probably be delighted that its techniques and practices were coming under closer examination. Others, perhaps HRM academics, may view evidence-based practice as simply another management fad. Box 9.5 provides an overview of the likely responses to evidence-based practice. Such responses imply that practitioners may believe that evidence-based practice (or a version of it) is already in place, that it is too difficult to apply or simply does not apply to this area, or that it would be welcomed.

Different practitioner groups are likely to react in different ways. For those who belong to professional bodies it is reasonable to assume that their response will, to some extent, be shaped by the reactions of the professional bodies to which they belong. In the case of the Institute of Personnel and Development, for example, as mentioned earlier, they do engage in limited sponsorship of research and may already feel their practice is, broadly speaking, evidence-based. For the occupational psychology division of the BPS (British Psychological Society) it also seems likely that they will assume that their practice is evidence-based. However,

> **Box 9.5: A summary of some possible responses to evidence-based practice in HRM**
>
> 'We're doing it, or enough of it already.'
> 'It takes a naïve and narrow view of evidence.'
> 'It takes a naïve view of how things really get done in organisations.'
> 'It's about time we did this.'
> 'It's not what the clients want.'
> 'There isn't enough evidence.'
> 'Who's going to pay for it?'
> 'It'd put me out of business.'
> 'What does it mean for my work?'
> 'It's politically unacceptable.'
> 'Organisations are just too complex to apply evidence to in this way.'

both these bodies are large and probably confident enough to take on or at least explore evidence-based practice as a means of enhancing their practices and professions.

For smaller-scale freelance consultants, who do not necessarily operate within such a context and proffer a wide range of interventions and techniques, evidence-based practice is likely to be viewed with some suspicion as a possible threat to the way in which they currently operate.

The reactions of relevant stakeholders will also be shaped by what they perceive the implications of evidence-based practice to be, as will be discussed next.

Some possible implications of evidence-based practice for HRM

As stated earlier, HRM practice has the potential to affect a substantial proportion of the population who are subjected to its techniques. Evidence-based practice in HRM is therefore likely to have implications for employees. More directly affected will be practitioners and academics. Each of these groups will be discussed in turn.

Implications for employees

Perhaps the most general implication is that employees can be more confident that the HRM techniques applied to them are likely to be more effective. Whether or not this is seen by employees to be of benefit will, of course, depend on whether or not perceived aims of those techniques are seen as benevolent or otherwise.

Given that evidence-based practice requires clear evidence and that within HRM a comprehensive or systematic evidence base does not yet exist, a further implication for employees is that they are likely to be subjected to considerably increased levels of assessment, measurement, and observation in relation to the introduction of new techniques, as practitioners and academics engage in research to collect further evidence and assessment to help guide choice of intervention. Employees can therefore expect to be subjected to greater levels of scrutiny or, as some may see it, surveillance.

At the same time, it may be that employees' views and attitudes towards new HRM initiatives will have to be more carefully taken into account by human resource managers and practitioners. The importance of local context in determining the success of HRM practices may mean that a much greater understanding of this is required both in choosing interventions and in their implementation. A further implication for employees and perhaps trades' unions is that they may experience greater levels of participation in decision-making.

Implications for HRM practitioners

The implications for practitioners are profound. While, as suggested earlier, we do not have good evidence about the way practitioners go about their work, it seems likely that the way in which evidence is used (if at all) cannot be compared with the use of evidence as advocated in evidence-based practice. The first and most general implication is therefore a marked shift in the way in which practitioners work and the increased use of both internal and external evidence. As indicated above, it appears that many HRM initiatives are not introduced on the basis of an assessment of needs, and in many cases existing evidence is either insufficient or inadequate. There would be a much greater emphasis for HRM practitioners on the routine collection and meaningful collation of internal data and in making initial assessments.

A second and related implication is for the training of practitioners. While some practitioners in this field, in particular occupational psychologists, should have the necessary expertise to critically appraise evidence, it appears as though the vast majority do not have such skills. This will mean that initial training will have to be very different: continuing professional development will have to move away from what often appears to be a somewhat instructional and technique-based approach, towards developing and maintaining the skills required for integrating the best available external evidence with the practitioner's own understanding and experience, in the manner outlined by Sackett *et al.* (1997) for medical practitioners. Skills in making internal assessments and evaluations of existing practices will also need to be developed. A third and related implication is that HRM practitioners may take on fewer fads and fashions, or at least be more healthily sceptical of their purported benefits.

A fourth implication, which is also an implication for academics, is that the nature of the relationship between practitioners and academics is likely to change as practitioners will have an increasing interest in research and in shaping the research agendas of academics.

Last, for external freelance practitioners or firms of HRM consultants, there will be considerable new demands to demonstrate that the techniques and practices they offer for sale or the services they provide are actually effective. For this group, this particular implication will be far-reaching and could result in fundamental changes to the HRM industry as a whole.

Implications for other organisational stakeholders

If HRM were to become more evidence-based, how would this impact on other organisational stakeholders? For managers and practitioners in other fields within the organisation it may mean that their own ways of working come to be viewed through the same evidence-based practice lens. Questions such as, Does it work? may then start to be applied to the activities of the marketing department, research and development, and so on. A culture of evidence-based practice may spread across other functions in organisations which have a significant HRM presence.

There are numerous other possible organisational stakeholders, including shareholders and, in the case of the public sector, civil servants, ministers, local counsellors and taxpayers. For each of these groups an important implication of evidence-based practice in HRM will be a raised awareness that the work of HRM practitioners could and should be more accountable. In other words, once the general principles of evidence-based practice are understood by these other stakeholders they are also likely to expect to see evidence for returns on the investment made in HRM – or at least evidence that funds are not being squandered on techniques of dubious efficacy.

Implications for academics and researchers

The most general implication is that the services of academics and researchers will be more in demand from practitioners. The initial training and continuing professional development of practitioners would require greater input from those with research expertise. Rather than a relatively small initial input about research methods, more time would be spent critically appraising evidence and using it in conjunction with other information, and this kind of training would continue throughout the career of a HRM practitioner.

Academics would be encouraged to translate their academic work into a more comprehensible format and be involved in the development of the HRM equivalents of the journal *Evidence-Based Mental Health*. At the present time no such journals exist for HRM practitioners.

One common problem for the HRM researcher is finding organisations that are willing to participate in research. An increased emphasis on research and evidence is likely to result in much easier access to organisations and even invitations to evaluate and assess HRM practice. A related implication concerns changes in funding. At the present time, HRM departments and HRM consultancies may be reluctant to fund research into their practices and policies as a possible outcome of the research is the discovery that they do not work. A move towards evidence-based practice would not entirely remove the fear of such an outcome but would at least make it more palatable and hence organisations may be far more willing to fund external research into what they do.

A further implication, as suggested before, is that the nature of the relationship between academics and practitioners is likely to change. Just as practitioners may become more immersed in research, so academics may find themselves closer than usual to organisational practices and HRM practitioners.

The vision of an evidence-based approach to HRM practice

To imagine what HRM would be like if it adopted evidence-based practice is something of an odd task. Sometimes the picture evoked is highly positive – if not rose-tinted: HRM practitioners, professional bodies, employees, and academics working together in order to ensure that HRM practices are effective, made accountable, and promote both individual and organisational effectiveness and well being. At other times, the image produced is less positive: one in which the importance of power, fad and pragmatism in determining what happens in HRM is recognised and where the somewhat naïve common-sense reasoning of evidence-based practice seems unlikely to hold much sway.

Many of the objections which will be raised to adoption of evidence-based practice are sound: very limited existing evidence; the complexities and difficulties of research in this field compared to some other fields – and in particular, looking at the effectiveness of HRM as a configuration or bundle of practices; the lack of funding; and perhaps most important, the huge shift in the thinking which will be required if evidence-based practice is to be adopted.

At the same time, it can be argued that HRM needs evidence-based practice – or at least something very much like it. Bold claims have already been made about the effectiveness of HRM on the basis of limited, though encouraging evidence. This evidence is very much top-down, largely concerning bundles of HRM practices, and does not yet appear to have had a major impact on the work of practitioners. If practitioners do not become more directly involved in using internal and external evidence, and significantly more evidence is not provided or made available about the effectiveness of specific practices (which is more relevant to the day-to-day work of practitioners), then it seems that the significant changes required to make HRM more effective and capable of adaptive change in the future will simply not happen. Evidence-based practice provides a possible starting point for achieving these aims.

References

Abrahamson E. (1996) Management fashion. *Academy of Management Review*, **21**, 254–85.

Aldag R.J. (1997) Moving sofas and exhuming woodchucks: on relevance, impact, and the following of fads. *Journal of Management Inquiry*, **6**, 8–16.

Barley S. & Kunda G. (1992) Design and devotion: surges of rational and normative ideologies of control in managerial discourse. *Administrative Science Quarterly*, **37**, 363–99.

Barrick M.R. & Mount M.K. (1991) The big five personality dimensions and job performance: a meta-analysis. *Personnel Psychology*, **44**, 1–26.

Becker B. & Gerhart B. (1996) The impact of human resource management on organisational performance: progress and prospects. *Academy of Management Journal*, **39**, 779–801.

Borman W.C., Hanson M.A. & Hedge J.W. (1997) Personnel selection. *Annual Review of Psychology*, **48**, 299–337.

Briner R.B. & Reynolds S. (1999) The costs, benefits, and limitations of organizational level stress interventions. *Journal of Organizational Behavior*, **20**, 647–64.

Clark T. & Salaman G. (1998) Telling tales: management gurus' narratives and construction of managerial identity. *Journal of Management Studies*, **35**, 137–61.

Department of Health (1998) *Working Together: Securing a Quality Workforce for the NHS*. DoH, Wetherby.

Dutton J.E. & Ashford S.J. (1993) Selling issues to top management. *Academy of Management Review*, **18**, 397–428.

Dutton J.E., Ashford S.J., O'Neill R.M., Hayes E. & Wierba E.E. (1997) Reading the wind: how middle managers assess the context for selling issues to top managers. *Strategic Management Journal*, **18**, 407–23.

Gill J. & Whittle S. (1993) Management by panacea: accounting for transience. *Journal of Management Studies*, **30**, 281–95.

Guest D.E. (1997) Human resource management and performance: a review and research agenda. *International Journal of Human Resource Management*, **8**, 263–76.

Harrison D.A. & Martocchio J.J. (1998) Time for absenteeism: a 20-year review of origins, offshoots, and outcomes. *Journal of Management*, **24**, 305–50.

Himmelfarb P.A. (1997) *Back to Basics: A Fad–Free Diet for Corporate Managers*. Philip Adam & Associates.

Huczynski A. (1993) *Management Gurus: What Makes Them and How to Become One*. Routledge, London.

Huselid M.A. (1995) The impact of human resource management practices on turnover, productivity, and corporate financial performance. *Academy of Management Journal*, **38**, 635–72.

Johns G. (1997) Contemporary research on absence from work: correlates, causes and consequences. In C.L. Cooper & I.T. Robertson (eds) *International Review of Industrial and Organisational Psychology: Volume 12*. Wiley, New York.

Legge K. (1995) *Human Resource Management: Rhetorics and Realities*. Macmillan, London.

Legge K. (1998) The morality of HRM. In C. Mabey, D. Skinner & T. Clark (eds) *Experiencing Human Resource Management*. Sage, London.

Locke E.A. & Latham G.P. (1990) Work motivation: the high performance cycle. In H-H.U. Kleinbeck, H. Quast & H. Hacker (eds) *Work Motivation*. Lawrence Erlbaum, New Jersey.

Mabey C., Clark T. & Skinner D. (1998) Getting the story straight. In C. Mabey, D. Skinner & T. Clark (eds) *Experiencing Human Resource Management*. Sage, London.

Miller P. (1996) Strategy and the ethical management of human resources. *Human Resource Management Journal*, **6**, 5–18.

Noe R.A. & Ford J.K. (1992) Emerging issues and new directions for training research. *Research in Personnel and Human Resource Management*, **10**, 345–84.

Porras J.I. & Robertson P.J. (1992) Organisational development: theory, practice, and research. In M.D. Dunnette & L.M. Hough (eds) *Handbook of Industrial and Organisational Psychology: Volume 3*. Consulting Psychologists Press, Palo Alto.

Rogers R. & Hunter J.E. (1992) Impact of management by objectives on organisational productivity. *Journal of Applied Psychology*, **76**, 322–36.

Rose M. (1998) *Industrial Behaviour: Theoretical Development Since Taylor* (3rd edition). Penguin, Harmondsworth.

Sackett D.L., Richardson W.S., Rosenburg W. & Haynes R.B. (1997) *Evidence-Based Medicine: How to Practice and Teach EBM*. Churchill Livingstone, London.

Shapiro E.C. (1995) *Fad Surfing in the Boardroom: Reclaiming the Courage to Manage in the Age of Instant Answers*. Capstone Publishing, Oxford.

Tannenbaum S.I., Salas E. & Cannon-Bowers J.A. (1996) Promoting team effectiveness. In M.A. West (ed.) *Handbook of Work Group Psychology*. Wiley, Chichester.

Tannenbaum S.I. & Yukl G. (1992) Training and development in work organisations. *Annual Review of Psychology*, **43**, 399–441.

Tett R.P., Jackson D.N. & Rothstein M. (1991) Personality measures as predictors of job performance: a meta-analytic review. *Personnel Psychology*, **44**, 407–740.

Truss C., Gratton L., Hope–Hailey V., McGovern P. & Stiles P. (1997) Soft and hard models of human resource management: a reappraisal. *Journal of Management Studies*, **34**, 53–73.

Williams, R.S. (1998) *Performance Management: Perspectives on Employee Performance*. International Thomson Business Press, London.

Chapter 10

A Critical Appraisal of Evidence-Based Practice

Liz Trinder

Introduction

In 1992 the Evidence-Based Medicine Working Group described the development of evidence-based medicine as 'profound enough that it can appropriately be called a paradigm shift'. Since that point evidence-based medicine has expanded rapidly from an idea into a movement, making a significant impact right across the broad field of health care to embrace, amongst others, dentistry, ophthalmology, pharmacology and toxicology, primary care, mental health, physiotherapy and occupational therapy, nursing, health promotion, purchasing policy and health management. Remarkably, too, the forward march of evidence-based practice has broken through the boundaries of the health disciplines and is beginning to impact on other disciplines, including education, social work and probation and human resource management, far beyond the medical origins of the movement. Evidence-based practice has, therefore, the potential to transform the distribution and delivery of public services both in the UK and elsewhere.

The aim of this chapter is to take stock of these developments and to critically appraise the relevance and helpfulness of evidence-based practice. The case study chapters (Chapters 3–9) offered an appraisal of evidence-based practice within individual disciplines. This chapter draws together the issues considered within the case study chapters and undertakes a broader examination of the strengths and weaknesses of evidence-based practice as a generic cross-disciplinary phenomenon. The chapter addresses two related questions:

- What are the strengths and weaknesses of evidence-based practice as a generic approach to practice?
- How useful and relevant is evidence-based practice across the range of disciplines that have adopted it, or might adopt it in future?

The chapter begins by identifying two opposing responses to evidence-based practice. It then moves on to consider the practical problems acknowledged by evidence-based practice enthusiasts before outlining the more conceptual difficulties highlighted by critics of evidence-based practice. The chapter concludes by identifying the challenges facing evidence-based practice.

Difficulties in critically appraising evidence-based practice

At the outset it has to be stated that there are no easy answers to the two questions this chapter is posing. The development and expansion of evidence-based practice has been marked by controversy, as will be evident from the preceding chapters. Evaluating the arguments and counter-arguments, claims and counter-claims of champions and critics is extremely difficult. There are a number of reasons why this is the case:

(1) Unmeasurability of evidence-based practice

Ironically, despite the centrality of measuring the effectiveness of interventions in evidence-based practice, it has not escaped the notice of either critics or champions that there is not, nor is likely to be, any empirical evaluation of the effectiveness of evidence-based practice itself (Rosenberg & Donald 1995). The lack of any empirical justification for the approach has meant that advocates have relied upon intuitive claims, whilst critics have countered on similar terms. Any critical appraisal of evidence-based practice can therefore only be based on opinion. The arguments in this chapter are, of course, no exception to this.

(2) Evolution across space

A further difficulty is that the nature of evidence-based practice is not constant across disciplines. It is clear from the case study chapters that evidence-based practice has been variously interpreted within particular disciplinary contexts (see also Chapter 1). There are differences between the population-based approach of evidence-based health care (Chapter 5) and the case-by-case approach of evidence-based primary care and mental health (Chapters 3 and 4). More significantly the approach begins to mutate in the accounts of evidence-based nursing with the introduction of qualitative research (Chapter 6), the top-down approach of evidence-based probation and education (Chapters 7 and 8) and the pluralistic interpretation within evidence-based social work (Chapter 7). The future development of evidence-based human resource management is as yet unclear (Chapter 9). Few of the models of practice outlined in the case study chapters mirror the classic approach to evidence-based medicine as set out in Chapter 2. We will discuss the merits and otherwise of the translation or evolution of evidence-based practice below, but the varied nature of the application of evidence-based practice does pose problems for evaluation.

(3) Distinguishing theory and practice: the 'straw man' argument

The third difficulty again concerns questions of definition. Enthusiasts often claim that criticisms of evidence-based practice, usually concerning the hierarchy of evidence and the role of consumers and professional expertise, rest upon a misinterpretation of evidence-based practice (see for example, Chapters 3 and 4). The frequently cited article by Sackett *et al.* (1996) on what evidence-based medicine is and is not, described 'a bottom-up approach that integrates the best external evidence with individual clinical expertise and patient-choice', and was explicitly designed to rebut what were seen as misplaced criticisms of 'cookbook' medicine. Despite the reassurances of enthusiasts it is apparent that the focus of the work to date has been on developing an evidence base and critical appraisal skills with meta-analysis and randomised controlled trials (RCTs) as the centerpieces. Comparatively little attention has yet been given to the questions of how to combine evidence with clinical experience or consumer perspectives. Lipman (Chapter 3 above) recognises that the textbook of Sackett *et al.* (1997) 'gives little detailed guidance on exactly how to do it, but [it is] unreasonable to assert that it cannot (and some would say should not) be done at all'. Whether or not the criticisms of evidence-based practice represent a misinterpretation of evidence-based practice, or alternatively a recognition of its weaknesses, can only be a matter of opinion at this early stage of development.

Champions and critics

For all the rapid successes of evidence-based practice, it is also evident that a consensus about the merits of evidence-based practice has not been forged, either within individual professions or across professions. The response to evidence-based practice can essentially be divided into two opposing camps of champions and critics, with little middle ground. In medicine the tireless enthusiasm for evidence-based practice of David Sackett and his colleagues has been met with often fierce opposition (e.g. Tanenbaum 1993; Carr-Hill 1995; Grahame-Smith 1995; *Lancet* 1995; Poly-chronis *et al.* 1966a,b; Smith & Taylor 1996; Hampton 1997; Shahar 1997). Similar exchanges are reported in each of the case study chapters above with the possible exception of the relatively undeveloped arena of human resource management. Indeed the perspectives of the contributors represented in this volume could equally be divided between champions and critics, again with little middle ground. The chapters by Gray, Geddes, Lipman and Briner would fit fairly readily within the evidence-based practice champions camp, with the remainder as critics.

There are, of course, difficulties with herding commentators into two binary opposites of champions and critics, not least of which is the tendency to freeze positions and prevent dialogue. Nonetheless the two positions do appear sufficiently distinct to provide a useful starting point for identifying and appraising viewpoints and potentially facilitating debate.

The champions

Amongst the champions there is a clear, coherent and consistent worldview or paradigm, fitting neatly into what Anthony Giddens identified as an approach of 'sustained optimism' (Chapter 1 above). For evidence-based practice champions there is an unshakeable belief in the capacity of science, and the rational and systematic application of science, to bring about effective, efficient and accountable practice (see Box 10.1). Furthermore, evidence-based practice is presented as a radical approach, where the neutrality of science and the transparency of the process provides the opportunity for both practitioners and consumers to participate. Knowledge, rather than authority or position, is privileged, and access to knowledge is available to anyone willing to learn the techniques or with access to the evidence.

For the champions, the major problems with evidence-based practice are essentially the structural and attitudinal barriers to its implementation, rather than any difficulties inherent in the approach. Over recent years, as we shall see below, some of the attention of the enthusiasts has shifted towards implementation, rather than mere advocacy, of evidence-based practice. The problems that are identified, which also represent the justification of the need for evidence-based practice, that is, difficulties in accessing evidence and limited appraisal skills, can also be largely solved by the tools of evidence-based practice. The development of evidence-based reviews, databases and guidelines, critical appraisal skills and a supporting infrastructure will all make the evidence-based practice process easier, providing of course that the approach is used systematically (Rosenberg & Donald 1995; Dawes 1996; and Chapter 4, this volume). Similarly evidence-based practice tools, including RCTs (randomised controlled trials) can be used to identify the effectiveness of different methods of implementing changes in practice. Thus evidence-based practice represents something like a total system, with an interlocking diagnosis, methodology and solution to the problem of the research–practice gap.

Box 10.1: Champions and critics of evidence-based practice

	Champions	*Critics*
General position on evidence-based practice	Essential and correct in principle and practice	Principle laudable but practice mistaken
Potential outcomes of evidence-based practice	(1) *Effective practice* with exclusion of ineffective and rapid adoption of effective interventions on a universal basis.	(1) *Unproven effectiveness of evidence-based practice* Possible exclusion of effective but unevidenced interventions. Possibility of 'formulaic' practice.
	(2) *Efficiency*: better use of scarce resources by practitioners and purchasers by ustilising only effective treatments.	(2) *Costs of implementing evidence-based practice*, direct and indirect financial and time costs of implementation, and unproven or incalculable savings.
	(3) *Value for money research* Better and more useful research and narrowing of research–practice gap.	(3) *Narrowing of research agenda*, reification of one form of research at the expense of other useful forms.
	(4) *Transparency and accountability of decision-making*	(4) *Hidden values* contained in the processes of research, summarising, and application, but not made explicit.
	(5) *Empowerment of practitioners* and ongoing self-directed learning of staff.	(5) *Threat to professional skills*, autonomy, decision-making, judgement dictated by narrow research agenda and managerialism.

Contd

Box 10.1 *Contd*

	(6) *Empowerment of consumers* within research and practice.	(6) *Incorporation of consumers* within professional agendas and processes.
	(7) *Enhanced multi-disciplinarity*	(7) *Enhancement of 'scientific' professions* and sub-disciplines at the expense of others and unhelpful convergence of professions.
Major problems of evidence-based practice	Barriers to implementation: • Low IT and critical appraisal skills • Limited infrastructure • Unwieldiness of and gaps in the evidence base • Time for practising evidence-based practice • Resistance to change.	Practical and technical difficulties with implementation. Scientific reductionism at the expense of other types of research evidence and other forms of knowledge and values. Mistaken certainty in dealing with complex issues.
Response to problems of evidence based practice	Problems can be addressed by evidence based practice methods and processes	Evidence-based practice does not provide a solution to the difficulties with evidence-based practice. Need to incorporate other types of evidence and knowledge and acknowledge weaknesses of evidence-based practice.
Centrality of evidence-based practice	New paradigm	Partial endorsement and incorporation as additional tool of greater or less utility within existing practice.

The critics

In contrast to the champions of evidence-based practice, the critics represent a much more disaggregated group. Indeed, part of the success of the evidence-based practice camp would appear to be related to the extent to which critics have failed to mount a coherent challenge or offer an alternative paradigm to the clarity of vision, degree of organisation and tightly focused approach of evidence-based practice. Whilst the enthusiasts might consider this to be a vindication of their approach, it is possible that the apparent floundering of the critics is simply a reflection of their own critique. Probably the only shared construct which unites the diverse band of critics is that the world of practice is more complex than that rendered by evidence-based practice, thereby largely precluding the construction of an alternative paradigm. This critique (see Box 10.1 for further details) essentially accuses evidence-based practice of an overly simplistic and reductionist approach, which fails to do justice to the inherent complexity of practice situations, and may mislead in the search for certainty. Although few, if any, would be prepared to reject evidence-based practice in its entirety, the utility and centrality to practice of evidence *per se* is greatly reduced compared to the total paradigm offered by evidence-based practice champions.

The opposing positions delineated in Box 10.1 are discussed in greater detail below. It is worth noting that for each claim for evidence-based practice, the opposing side has a rebuttal. The table should be read from both left-to-right and right-to-left.

The remainder of this chapter focuses in more detail on some of the issues identified in Box 10.1. The discussion is divided into two parts: the following section identifies some of the technical or practical problems with evidence-based practice that have been acknowledged by both champions and critics. We then turn towards some of the more fundamental issues raised by critics but largely rebutted by champions of evidence-based practice.

Practical problems with evidence-based practice

Is there evidence available?

A frequent observation made by the evidence-based practice enthusiasts is that there is simply too much research to manage, much of it of poor quality or of limited relevance, resulting in practitioners being unable to identify readily the current best evidence. This complaint is echoed across the range of activities represented in this book. One of the advantages of the evidence-based practice movement is the potential that it provides for systematisation of the knowledge base within individual disciplines, for regular updating of the knowledge base as well as for the capacity to identify and fill gaps through, for example, the NHS Health Technology Assessment Programme.

It is clear however that generating an evidence base will be an enormous undertaking. Although there is a surfeit of evidence in some areas, it is clear that for many areas of practice the problem is one of scarcity rather than voluminosity; the existing research base is unevenly distributed. Within medicine, Culpepper & Gilbert (1999) argue that there is more evidence available within medical specialties than in general medical practice where most interventions have a limited evidence base. The case study chapters on education, social work, human resource management and nursing also indicate how little research there is at the top of the hierarchy of evidence. Without evidence-based practice it is unlikely that these gaps would be filled; however, even with the mechanisms in place to identify gap areas it would require a considerable redirection of research effort and funding to begin to plug them (see Box 10.2).

Box 10.2: The availability of evidence	
Problems	• availability of high-quality evidence • uneven distribution of high-quality evidence.
Advantages of evidence-based practice	• identification of gap areas • mechanisms to address gaps.
Difficulties of evidence-based practice	• differential researchability by area • uneven funding mechanisms • possible skew of interventions towards evidence rather than effectiveness.
Challenges	• ensuring the development of an evenly distributed evidence base.

Even with a redirection of effort and funding, it is apparent that some areas are inherently more researchable than others, particularly if the aim is to achieve high-level evidence. The skewing of the research base in medicine towards some specialties rather than general practice, and in, for example, human resource management towards individual rather than organisational interventions (see Chapter 9), reflect genuine methodological difficulties which are not easily surmounted.

In the meantime the uneven distribution of the evidence base not only constrains the full development of evidence-based practice, it also has implications for what services may be purchased or provided. It is possible that some effective interventions will be discounted or rejected, not because they are ineffective, but because they cannot yet (or ever) produce sufficient high quality of evidence. On this point Kerridge *et al.* (1998) warn that the distinction between a therapy 'without substantial evidence' and 'without substantial value' might easily be elided. Indeed it is clear that evidence-based purchasing decisions are already impacting on what will, and crucially what will not, be funded. In 1997, Lambeth, Southwark and Lewisham Health Authority withdrew funding for homeopathic treatment on the grounds that there was not enough strong evidence to support its use (Wise 1997).

One of the strengths of evidence-based practice is the opportunity it affords to directly compare the effectiveness of different interventions. However, one of the issues that is yet to be resolved is how to ensure that different interventions, and different professional groups, are able to compete on a level playing field. Where two or more different disciplines are occupying the same terrain, as in the case of mental health (see Chapter 4), this issue becomes particularly visible. As John Geddes recognises, there is a danger that the relative importance (and purchasing) of drugs and talking cures might well be skewed by the greater volume of evidence available for drugs-based therapies. Although evidence-based practice might empower some professional groupings, Lipman (see Chapter 3), for example, makes a strong case for GPs, there are questions about whether each profession is equally capable of enhancement given the unequal distribution of evidence.

Can practice be changed?

For the champions, the major problems with evidence-based practice are the largely technical or structural barriers frustrating its implementation (Rosenberg & Donald 1995; Dawes 1996; Chapter 5, this volume; Chapter 4, this volume; Haines & Haines 1998). The conclusions from the Frontline Project (Donald 1998) illustrate some of these difficulties. The project was designed to examine the feasibility of introducing evidence-based medicine methods into routine clinical practice involving 20 hospital teams. The overall conclusion was that the introduction of evidence-based practice was both possible and desirable but that significant difficulties remained. The major problems identified were:

- inadequate access to information, particularly the difficulties in getting Internet-linked computers on wards available for all staff, and with access to full-text articles
- lack of relevant evidence
- low level of computer and critical appraisal skills, and limited time available to acquire them
- medical and nursing hierarchies
- perceived threats to medical autonomy.

Box 10.3: Can evidence-based practice be implemented?	
Identified problems	• gap between evidence and practice • difficulties in introducing evidence-based practice in projects and generalising • absence of 'magic bullets' for effective dissemination and implementation.
Information deficit model (champions)	Solutions are technical and structural: • hardware and software • IT and critical appraisal skills training • development of an evidence base.
Complex model (critics)	Solutions as above, and: • local negotiations and trust building • effective involvement of practitioners, managers and consumers • multifaceted implementation strategies • attention to knock-on effects of introducing change in practice on other services.
Challenges	Introducing, generalising and sustaining change

The principal problem identified is principally informational, neatly meshing with the rationale for evidence-based practice, as the report concludes:

> 'the project revealed that in almost all cases, the most formidable barriers to the use of evidence in clinical practice were structural and logistical problems, such as the complete absence in most settings of updated databases of research findings, and lack of time or space in which to train clinicians with new skills, rather than behavioural problems of clinicians, as much of the current literature would suggest'.
>
> (Donald 1998: 4)

The recommended solutions also draw upon the tools of evidence-based practice, that is, tackling access to information by providing hardware and databases including the Cochrane Library, IT and critical appraisal training and alerting research funders about gaps in the evidence base. Interestingly the attitudinal problems identified by the project – occupational hierarchies and perceived threats to autonomy – are also provided with informational solutions, that is joint training and information about other occupations, and waiting for reluctant participants to see the value of evidence-based practice in action (and see Gray, Chapter 5).

The enduring belief amongst evidence-based practice champions is that the principal barrier to evidence-based practice is an information deficit

(Marteau *et al.* 1998). If practitioners can access and apply the right information and discard the wrong information then evidence-based practice can be implemented and practice will be enhanced. However this rather optimistic or naïve assumption that making evidence available is sufficient to ensure its utilisation is being challenged by other studies of implementation (NHS Centre for Reviews and Dissemination 1999: 2). A growing body of research is indicating that although evidence-based practice enthusiasts (amongst others) are correct in identifying the limited extent to which practitioners draw upon research, their solutions for tackling it underestimate the complexity and extent of the task of introducing change.

Although there remain difficulties in disseminating information, it is also clear that the obstacles to implementation go beyond information deficits, that there is a distinction between dissemination and implementation. A review of seven studies of critical appraisal training, for example, indicated that medical students experienced a substantial increase in knowledge of critical appraisal, although the impact on junior doctors was very much smaller. There was, however, no evidence that the training was translated into actual changes in clinical practice for junior doctors, or that the knowledge gains of undergraduates would be sustained into practice (Norman & Shannon 1998). A review of continuing medical educational strategies (including courses and conferences) similarly found little effect (Davis *et al.* 1995). Reviews have found that the simple circulation of guidelines alone (i.e. passive dissemination) is ineffective without an active dissemination strategy (NHS Centre for Reviews and Dissemination 1994). Nor are there any 'magic bullets' in terms of particularly effective single strategies for dissemination (Oxman *et al.* 1995). A recent summary of a range of reviews of broad strategies (including education and guidelines) targeted interventions to change specific behaviours (including preventive care and prescribing) and specific interventions (including educational materials, educational outreach, audit and feedback, and reminders) concludes that:

> 'Most interventions are effective under some circumstances, none is effective under all circumstances ... Multi-faceted interventions targeting different barriers to change are more likely to be effective than single interventions'.
>
> (NHS Centre for Review and Dissemination 1999: 7)

Demonstration projects examining the implementation of evidence-based practice illustrate some of the challenges involved. The PACE (Promoting Action on Clinical Effectiveness) programme consisted of 16 local projects, each working on a specific single clinical topic (Dunning *et al.* 1997). The FACTS (Framework of Appropriate Care Throughout Sheffield) project was designed to work on three linked coronary heart disease interventions in general practice (Eve *et al.* 1997). Like the Frontline Project, both PACE and FACTS indicate that progress towards evidence-based practice can be achieved. They also indicate how complex and difficult change is. Although acknowledging the role of technical barriers to information, the focus is much more on the interpersonal and organisational processes involved, emphasising the need for prior and ongoing localised negotiations and discussion in order to secure support and commitment:

> 'The bad news is that there are no magic bullets, no quick-fit tool boxes packed with nifty tricks to achieve this. Instead there is the much more complicated business of listening to people, solving the real world problems they tell you are inhibiting them and inspiring them to change. Multi-faceted programmes built around these principles, tailored to specific purposes, fitted to particular circumstances and purveyed by agencies capable of building trust and credibility are likely to generate real change'.
>
> (Eve *et al.* 1997: 40)

The findings from the PACE project also emphasise that the focus of change efforts must be broader than resting with individual clinicians. Successful and sustained change must involve the active input of managers, policy-makers, patients and clinicians, as well as effective working relationships between them. The knock-on effects of changes in clinical practice, for example changes in GP referral rates, will also require broader changes in service provision (Dunning *et al.* 1997).

Implementing change therefore requires consideration of organisational, economic and community environments as well as the knowledge, attitudes and beliefs of individuals, and will involve detailed analysis and planning and a range of different implementation techniques and strategies (NHS Centre for Reviews and Dissemination 1999). It should be emphasised that Frontline, FACTS, and PACE were modest projects, seeking change within a small number of wards or in single districts, and for FACTS and PACE, on single clinical topics where strong evidence existed. Translating the achievements of individual projects into change throughout the health care field, and then sustaining change, will be an enormous task, not least in terms of time and money. Rosenberg & Donald (1995b) suggest that the benefits of creating an evidence-based infrastructure might well outweigh the cost. At present this can only be speculative given that the gains are incalculable, as indeed are the full costs of implementing evidence-based practice.

To date the bulk of research, and the discussion here, has focused exclusively on health care, particularly medicine. At present we can only speculate about the prospects for implementation of evidence-based practice elsewhere. On the positive side, many of the lessons from health care implementation, including the major research programme on implementation currently being undertaken by the Department of Health, may be capable of being generalised elsewhere. On the other hand, it would appear unlikely that implementation of evidence-based practice will be any easier outside of health, where the research infrastructure and skills base is, if anything, even more limited, and evidence-based initiatives are both less numerous and less advanced. The prospects for human resource management are even harder to read. Within the health service the organisational framework for evidence-based practice which already exists is likely to prove a significant resource; in the private sector the lack of a coherent organisational and professional framework may well frustrate efforts to develop an evidence-based practice framework (Chapter 9, this volume).

The task becomes even greater bearing in mind the requirement to base practice on the *current* best evidence. Even with the inbuilt updating process of the Cochrane Collaboration there remains a time lag between the appearance of new and potentially conflicting evidence and the updating of reviews (Griffiths 1995; and see reply of Rosenberg & Donald 1995a). This exchange between Griffiths, and Rosenberg and Donald justifies the regular revisions undertaken by the Cochrane Collaboration, but, for the foreseeable future, it is unlikely to be practical in other areas.

It is worth noting at this point that many of the implementation projects as well as the initiatives described in the case study chapters focus on the implementation of guidelines, rather than individual practitioners utilising the full-blown five-step model of question, search, appraise, apply and evaluate for individual cases outlined in Chapter 2 above. There are several possible reasons for this. Time and skills appear to be significant factors. Lipman (see Chapter 3) notes the preference of GPs for research digests rather than for developing their own critical appraisal skills.

Relying on guidelines, however, can only be a partial solution to implementation problems. Good guidelines will be highly specific rather than of wide applicability. Thus Lipman (Chapter 3, this volume) notes that introducing five evidence-based guidelines in general practice would apply to fewer than 3% of cases being dealt with. The other problem is that a guidelines-led approach risks providing a blanket solution to individual problems. There is some indication that in probation and education the focus at present is on a top-down and fairly prescriptive approach to implementation of evidence-based practice, led by managers and policy-makers rather than the professionally led origins of evidence-based medicine (see Trinder, Chapter 7, Hammersley, Chapter 8, this volume). Whilst this may short circuit some of the difficulties with implementation, the indications from projects like FACTS would suggest that change is unlikely to occur without building local coalitions of support amongst practitioners.

The lessons from studies of implementation indicate that the identification of the problem of evidence-based enthusiasts is essentially correct, as is the identification of the technical and informational barriers to implementation. However, the solutions presented appear increasingly at odds with the evidence presented from implementation studies. Implementing evidence-based practice will be a massive, lengthy and complex undertaking requiring much more than the simple provision of information and training in its appraisal. To some extent the tools of evidence-based practice will assist with this, the steady development of an evidence-based infrastructure will facilitate the process, as will research into different methods of implementation. They are insufficient by themselves, however.

Critics might point out too that what the studies of the implementation of evidence-based practice have also indicated is that social or non-biological interventions by professionals (of which interventions to implement evidence-based practice are just another example), are not easily reduced to numerical data of what works. The recent *Effective Health Care Bulletin, Getting Evidence into Practice*, concludes that RCTs are an important, but not a sufficient, means of providing indicators of the relative effectiveness of different interventions, and calls for 'a mixture of both qualitative and quantitative methods in order to assess not just the effectiveness of interventions but gain understanding of the process of professional behaviour change' (NHS Centre for Reviews and Dissemination 1999: 14). These methodological issues are considered in the following section.

Conceptual problems with evidence-based practice

In the previous section we looked at some of the technical difficulties associated with evidence-based practice. The difficulties with establishing an evidence base and implementing change are acknowledged by evidence-based practice enthusiasts, indeed much of the rationale for the need for evidence-based practice is predicated on that very basis. The argument of the champions is that it will be largely persistence and the tools of evidence-based practice that will be able to break down these barriers. Clearly not everybody agrees with this analysis. In this section we will draw together some of the more fundamental criticisms of evidence-based practice raised earlier in this book. The arguments of the critics go beyond the practical question of whether or not evidence-based practice can be implemented, and highlight what are seen as fundamental errors in the model. For the critics, evidence-based practice is seen as an incomplete or a reductionist approach to practice, based on 'scientism' rather than science, producing partial and potentially misleading understandings of real-world situations. In this volume, the critics are largely represented within the chapters on nursing, social work and probation and education, although similar questions are raised elsewhere within medicine.

To simplify what are often complex debates we will consider three questions in turn:

(1) Can 'evidence' be trusted?
(2) Does evidence-based practice produce knowledge that is useful to practitioners?
(3) Can evidence-based practice incorporate, or do justice to, other forms of knowledge, including practitioner experience and consumer perspectives?

Can the evidence be trusted? Is objective data possible?

Evidence-based practice is premised on the availability of high-quality evidence that is valid, reliable and free of bias. Gray (Chapter 5 above), for example, argues that the emergence of evidence-based decision-making has ensured a distinction between propositions supported by evidence and those supported by personal experience, values or resources. The methodological criteria that are advocated within evidence-based practice, particularly via the Cochrane Collaboration, are explicitly designed to distinguish findings of high-quality studies from invalid or unreliable data of poorly conducted research studies. In theory, the undoubted rigour of these procedures, and the regular updating of reviews, should produce data that can be trusted and are worthy of the title 'evidence'.

Critics, however, continue to raise questions about how trustworthy and unbiased evidence can be. The analysis ranges from technical questions about specific techniques to more fundamental concerns about the possibility of objective knowledge (see Box 10.4).

Box 10.4: Can the evidence be trusted?	
Enthusiasts	• rigorous adherence to methodological criteria ensures high-quality valid and reliable evidence.
Critics	• problems with meta-analysis • allegiance bias • inevitability of interpretation in the production of evidence.
Challenges	• acknowledging uncertainty in evidence.

Meta-analysis

Meta-analysis is vitally important within evidence-based practice as a component of systematic reviews, located at the top of the hierarchy of evidence (see Box 4.4, Chapter 4; Gray 1997). The rationale for meta-analysis is that it provides a larger sample than is generally possible within individual randomised trials and that the inclusion of a number of studies irons out the possibility of chance effects within individual studies. There

are a number of identified difficulties with meta-analysis, including publication bias towards positive trials and duplicate publishing of the same
trial data under different authors, both of which potentially skew the
results of a meta-analysis. The evidence-based practice movement has
done much to highlight these problems and to take steps to remedy them.
However, problems remain. Discrepancies have been found between the
results of meta-analyses of smaller studies and later single large RCTs
addressing the same question (Greenhalgh 1997; Naylor 1997). As Naylor
comments:

> 'meta-analyses may generate misleading results by ignoring meaningful
> heterogeneity among studies, entrenching the biases in individual studies, and
> introducing further biases through the process of finding studies and selecting
> results to be pooled'.
>
> (Naylor 1997)

A graphical funnel plot technique may be of assistance in identifying some
misleading meta-analyses, though not all. Using the technique Egger *et al.*
(1997) suggest that five reviews within the Cochrane database of systematic
reviews were potentially misleading. Whilst Naylor (1997) and Egger and
Smith (1997) would concur that meta-analysis would generally be superior
to narrative reviews, neither would view meta-analysis as infallible.

Allegiance bias

Research on effectiveness is inherently political, with practitioners and
researchers attached to a particular profession, or preferred method of
intervention, and potentially having a lot to lose. This holds for both public
sector and private sector organisations, whether in the form of drugs
companies or human resource management consultancies (see Chapter 9,
this volume). This, of course, provides much of the rationale for the
attempts to exclude bias within evidence-based practice, but it does also
pose one of its major challenges. It is not at all clear that the mechanisms
put in place will eliminate allegiance bias amongst researchers. To date, the
debate about allegiance bias has probably advanced furthest in the field of
mental health, yet few solutions are apparent.

Uncertainty and interpretation

The last issue to look at here is the place of interpretation within evidence.
Champions of evidence-based practice emphasise the importance of
uncertainty, however this is framed in terms of not being required to know
all the answers but having the ability to find out (e.g. Rosenberg & Donald
1995; see also Chapter 5, this volume). Whilst there is a sense that evidence

is provisional, and will be updated in the light of findings from new studies, there is a reluctance to acknowledge uncertainty about the evidence itself, by exploring how the process of building evidence is shaped by values and interpretation.

One of the criticisms of evidence-based practice is that decisions about what to research, how to research it, and what to measure, involve value judgements (or meta-theories) which are not always recognised or acknowledged. At the broadest level, for example, Gray (see Chapter 5 above) refers to (but does not endorse) the argument that focusing on quality in health care may deflect attention from the relationship between poverty and health. The quantitative foundation of evidence-based practice also requires the selection of outcomes that are measurable, thus including some questions and excluding others. Hammersley (Chapter 8 above) argues that centring on effectiveness involves a focus on measurable outcomes at the expense of other important educational goals. In probation the focus has shifted away from the socio-economic situation of probationers to their cognitions, partly reflecting the greater ease with which the latter can be researched by RCTs (see Chapter 7). The process of selection of outcome measures is, of course, a highly political process given that different individuals will have different perspectives on what outcomes are important (see Smith & Cantley 1985; Hammersley, Chapter 8). Whilst organisations like the Cochrane Collaboration have attempted to incorporate consumer perspectives, it is clear that the extent to which these have impacted upon the process and outcomes of review groups is variable (Bastian 1994; Cochrane Collaboration Consumer Network 1998).

Finally, it is important to recognise that the process of reviewing evidence also involves interpretation at each stage. The Cochrane Collaboration has developed rigorous processes for review, but the process can never be entirely technical or devoid of interpretation, in, for example, what studies are included, how they are interpreted and how they are summarised. The Collaboration attempts to make these decisions as transparent as possible and therefore open to challenge. The epistemological framework of researchers may, however, preclude awareness of particular biases. Hilda Bastian comments that incorporating consumer perspectives:

> 'will be especially difficult in the Cochrane Collaboration, where many researchers' claims of objectivity in their analyses suggest that they are unaware of the value-laden elements of what they do at so many steps along the way. Consumers and professionals may well see "threats to validity" in completely different places'.

> (Bastian 1994)

The work of the evidence-based practice movement has highlighted the issue of quality in research. The Cochrane Collaboration in particular has taken major steps towards refining rigorous procedures for assessing methodological quality and eliminating bias. Major challenges remain, however. First, achieving this level of methodological sophistication across the whole field of professional interventions will be an enormous task. Second, as critics have pointed out, the claims for objectivity implicit in the term evidence may well be overstated and mask hidden assumptions and values. The challenge therefore will be to reflexively acknowledge this degree of uncertainty rather than reifying evidence, whilst avoiding the alternative trap of relativism.

Can evidence be applied? Does it provide useful knowledge?

Aside from trustworthiness, the other required aspect of evidence is that research is useful or relevant for practice (see Chapter 2 above). It is unquestionable that evidence-based practice, and associated developments, have produced knowledge which is useful if not vital for practitioners and consumers. The use of aspirin after myocardial infarction is a prime example. However, critics continue to raise questions about how applicable much evidence is in real-life practice situations. These criticisms centre, in particular, on the role of RCTs and meta-analyses, and are most strongly articulated, although not confined to, areas of practice where the interventions are non-biological (see Box 10.5).

Box 10.5: Can the evidence be applied?	
Enthusiasts	• evidence-based practice procedures involve distilling high-quality evidence of direct relevance for practice.
Critics	• aggregate data • internal versus external validity • identifying causal mechanisms.
Challenges	• developing research designs facilitating application of research • more attention to issues of using research in practice.

Aggregate and averaged effects

One of the commonest questions raised of evidence-based practice is the extent to which evidence generated from aggregate populations can be applied to individuals (e.g. Sweeney 1996; and see Chapter 2 above). Whilst the evidence of average effects can facilitate decisions about the overall purchasing or distribution of services (in situations where the evidence does support clear recommendations), it is less easily applied to the individuals with whom practitioners deal. The averaged-out effect identified by an RCT contains individuals for whom the intervention produced an average, an above average and a below average effect. It is not clear therefore whether or not a particular individual will experience a benefit, a harm or no effect from an intervention.

Internal versus external validity

Decisions about the application of aggregate data to individuals may well be further complicated by the apparent conflict between maximising the internal validity of a study and its external validity or applicability in practice (e.g. Knottenerus *et al.* 1997; see also Geddes, Chapter 3 above). Black (1996) identifies three threats to the generalisability or external validity of RCTs in health care:

(1) *Professionals who participate may be unrepresentative* (of the broader population of professionals): as enthusiasts, innovators, highly experienced, or experts.
(2) *Patients may be atypical*: restrictive exclusion criteria to ensure internal validity mean that patients within trials might represent a small and unrepresentative proportion of all patients to whom the intervention might be seen as suitable. Older people, women, non-English speakers are typically excluded, as are those with co-morbidity.
(3) *Treatment may be atypical.*

Thus RCTs provide an indication of the *efficacy* of an intervention under the most favourable circumstances, rather than its *effectiveness* in everyday situations. There is no guarantee that studies of effectiveness and efficacy will produce similar conclusions (see Chapter 2 above). Black (1996) notes that the issue of external validity has not been addressed as a criteria for judging the quality of trials. This remains a challenge that has not been addressed so far by evidence-based practice enthusiasts, nor has much attention been given to efficacy studies.

Generalising or applying the results of RCTs in *social* or non-biological interventions appears to pose particular challenges. Here, the far less uniform characteristics of providers, settings and patients may be linked to outcomes in ways that can be imperfectly measured or understood, in contrast to the generally more uniform effect of purely biological interventions (Black 1996; Sweeney 1996; Sheldon *et al.* 1998). This is further compounded by the frequent lack of easily identifiable diagnostic categories in many areas of practice (McGuire *et al.* 1997). Similarly, whilst RCTs typically focus on single issues, many of the individuals seen by practitioners typically have a more complex range of problems (e.g. see van Weel 1996; Knottnerus *et al.* 1997; and Chapters 6 and 7 above). The complexity of individual cases is not ignored by evidence-based practice but still remains undeveloped, particularly in interventions beyond biological processes. It is unclear whether the mathematical gymnastics required to produce a composite NNT from separate trials for patients with multiple conditions (as in one reported case example of a woman with hypertension) (see Glasziou *et al.* 1998), will find widespread endorsement, or be technically feasible in most situations.

Identifying causal mechanisms

A further limitation of RCTs, particularly in social interventions, is that although useful for identifying outcomes, they offer limited purchase on what the precise mechanisms are that generate effects. Understanding *why* an intervention works, or does not work with specific individuals or groups, is a crucial means of tailoring interventions to specific situations. John Geddes' case study of models of community care provides a good example of the difficulties in isolating causal mechanisms (see Chapter 3 above). It is not clear, as Geddes acknowledges, to what extent data from studies of service provision conducted in the USA can be generalised to the UK. In particular, it is not clear precisely what aspects of different models of community care, in what combinations, actually make a difference to outcomes (see also Chapters 7, 8 and 9 for the difficulties in identifying causal effects).

Without an understanding of what mechanisms are important, the application of evidence is likely to be a blunt instrument. Sub-group analyses can be used to gain some understanding of what is occurring within the 'black box' of an intervention. However, these are not often undertaken, and the selection of measurable variables such as age and gender may or may not be the relevant or important variables. To date, evidence-based practice has largely consigned qualitative research into a preliminary hypothesis-generating role or into identifying consumer perspectives. It may now be time, as is happening with research on the effectiveness of studies to implement evidence-based practice, to incorporate qualitative and other non-RCT quantitative studies into research on the *process* of effectiveness, particularly where the interventions are themselves processes.

To date, limited attention has been paid to how evidence can be applied in practice. This discussion has highlighted the limitations of data derived from RCTs and suggested that other research designs may well be required to sharpen up the broad brush strokes provided by RCTs. The application of evidence, however, also has to be understood in relation to other knowledge, including professional experience and consumer preferences and values. These are considered in the next section.

Can evidence-based practice incorporate, or be integrated with, other forms of knowledge and values?

Evidence-based practice is a linear and rational approach to decision-making based on quantified data, aiming to establish practice on a scientific basis. Not surprisingly, critics of evidence-based practice have expressed concern that the dominance or centrality of science will devalue or exclude other forms of knowledge and values. The frequently cited definition of evidence-based medicine by Sackett *et al.* (1996) refers to the integration of evidence with clinical experience and patient preferences and values. This final section examines the practical and ontological issues involved in combining different types of knowledge, considering in turn the role of professional experience and understanding, theory and consumer values and preferences (see Box 10.6).

Box 10.6: The place of other forms of knowledge and values

Enthusiasts	Evidence-based practice integrates best available evidence with: • individual clinical expertise (proficiency and judgement) • patient (consumer) values and preferences.
Critics	• focus on the measurable, devaluing or rationalisation of other forms of knowledge • limited focus on the art of practice • possible downgrading of patient or consumer stories • exclusion of theory.
Challenges	Ensuring other forms of knowledge are incorporated fully into the model, and on their own terms.

The 'art' of practice

One argument of the critics is that evidence-based practice over-emphasises the importance or relevance of scientific evidence at the expense of professional experience, knowledge and reflection. For the critics the role of science is inherently limited in certain professions. Blomfield & Hardy and Hammersley in particular distinguish between what Schon calls the 'hard, high ground' and technical rationality of research and the indeterminate and unpredictable 'swamplands' of practice in nursing and education (see also Sweeney's 1996 discussion of general practice). Thus, whilst research evidence has a place, the argument is that what most of what many professions do is practical rather than technical work, which is not easily or appropriately standardised, either in the research process or in practice (see Hammersley, Chapter 8, this volume).

The second aspect of this argument is that the focus on scientifically defined interventions appears to shift the focus away from the caring, emotional and supportive aspects of professional work transforming the nature of the profession, an issue which is of concern in nursing (see Chapter 6 above) and has been extensively explored in general practice (e.g. Sweeney 1996; Sullivan 1996; Jacobson *et al.* 1997). To date there has been little work done on identifying the balance or weighting of evidence and experience.

Empowering consumers?

It is apparent that the agendas, priorities, interpretations and values of consumers are often at variance with those of professionals. Professionals can often have a limited understanding of consumers' perspectives or concerns, in health (e.g. Entwistle *et al.* 1998a) or other disciplines such as social work (Mayer & Timms 1970). In some areas of practice reluctant consumers may not even subscribe to the goal of more effective practice (Briner, see Chapter 9, this volume). Nor have researchers been particularly effective in addressing issues that are of importance to consumers. Entwistle *et al.* (1998b: 216) note the limited amount of evidence that incorporates outcomes that matter to patients. Bastian (1994) similarly identifies how little issues of significance to women, such as pain and discomfort, are included in research reviewed in the Cochrane pregnancy and childbirth database.

We noted in Chapter 1 the general societal shift towards consumer empowerment. The evidence-based practice movement shares this focus on the consumer; indeed, much of the rationale of the movement is that more effective and safer practice is in the interests of the consumer. However, evidence-based practice also seeks the *involvement* of consumers within the process of generating evidence, and in the decision-making process.

Probably the most well-known example of involving consumers within the process of assembling evidence is the involvement of users within Cochrane Collaboration review groups, supported by the Cochrane Consumer Network. Although the initiative is to be welcomed, it does also highlight the challenges involved in bringing together two very different perspectives, with different world-views, experiences, priorities and cultures (e.g. see Cochrane Collaboration Consumer Network 1998). Nor is it clear the extent to which consumer perspectives can fully inform a largely scientific process. A study by Kelson on the use of patient-defined outcomes within 33 Cochrane review groups found that four groups were 'committed in practice', 22 were 'committed in theory' and six were 'unconvinced' (cited in Meredith 1998).

The responsiveness of evidence-based practice to consumer concerns is somewhat contradictory. Whilst aspects of the model invite consumer participation, central features of the process inhibit participation. The priorities and sources of authority of scientific and consumer perspectives are likely to differ in key ways, and it appears difficult to focus on the outcomes that matter to patients, particularly within the context of RCTs (see Box 10.7). Whilst the authority of consumer voices is elicited and valued within evidence-based practice, other aspects of the model, particularly the hierarchy of evidence, may exclude or diminish the extent to which these can be incorporated.

Box 10.7: Scientific and consumer perspectives		
	Scientific perspectives	*Consumer perspectives*
Prime source of evidence	Hierarchy of evidence with opinion at the bottom, RCT and meta-analysis at the top	Centrality of experience, principally qualitative
Level of analysis	• evidence from aggregate populations • selected outcome indicators.	• evidence from individualised experiences • holistic real-life experiences.
Principle mode of operation	Reason	Emotion

In terms of decision-making, a number of studies have found benefits in outcomes for patient involvement in health decisions (Coulter *et al.* 1999) and in other areas of practice (Thoburn *et al.* 1995). Again, it is unclear whether evidence-based practice will facilitate or inhibit this process.

One potential danger of evidence-based practice is that the focus shifts towards questions of what is to be done and away from hearing people's stories. A number of commentators have expressed concern that the focus on doing shifts attention away from the essential prior step of feeling and understanding. Sweeney (1996: 76), for example, argues that 'The consultation in general practice is not simply a place where a patient seeks scientific answers to questions' but is also about coming to understand an illness, emotionally as well as rationally. This process of understanding, or telling one's story, is not only vital for the individual, it is probably the most important source of evidence in many cases in terms of identifying courses of action (Sweeney 1996; Sullivan & MacNaughton 1996).

Identifying means by which consumers can be informed about treatment options is also problematic. Professionals are in a powerful position in relation to consumers, and how information is framed, as well as what information is included, may significantly impact upon consumers' own decisions (Entwistle *et al.* 1998b). The additional authority conveyed by the term evidence or discussion of methodological quality may complicate this further. Furthermore Entwistle *et al.* (1998b: 222) warn of the dangers of leading or forcing people into a rational decision-making process, which could preclude people making decisions based on their own values and priorities. Considerable time and effort will be required to facilitate consumer involvement, and must be tailored to the needs and decision-making styles of individuals, and go beyond the mere provision of information (Entwistle *et al.* 1998b).

The role of theory

The role of theory is the other source of knowledge with uncertain status within evidence-based practice. It is interesting to note that the relevance of theories of change have been highlighted in discussions of the implementation of evidence-based practice (e.g. Grol 1997; NHS Centre for Reviews and Dissemination 1999). The further development of evidence-based practice will require consideration of the role of theory.

Challenges

Evidence-based practice is an empirically led strategy that has yet to identify how other forms of knowledge can inform or be integrated within the model. It remains unclear how consumer preferences and evidence can be combined (Entwistle *et al* 1998b), nor is the relationship between clinical experience and theory particularly developed. The risk is that the importance of these other forms of knowledge is diminished by a focus on a particular scientific form of knowledge. At present this aspect of the model remains under-developed in comparison with the clarity of the processes for developing an evidence base. Aside from the Sackett *et al.* definition of evidence-based practice, little attention has been given to this other than a small number of descriptive case studies (Glasziou *et al.* 1998; Godlee 1998).

The challenges ahead

It is ironic that such a scientific and rational project as evidence-based practice tends to provoke intense feelings. The debate about evidence-based practice has been polarised between the champions who have been reluctant to accept any criticisms of the model, and the critics who have been reluctant to accept any advantages of the approach. From its beginnings evidence-based medicine has attracted criticism, and the expansion of evidence-based practice into new fields has brought further protests echoing similar, if not heightened, concerns as the original critics.

Evidence-based practice remains in the early stages of development in medicine, and even more so elsewhere. To date the focus of attention has been on advocacy for the model and developing systems for generating evidence. As evidence-based practice develops, however, a number of cracks are beginning to show and its claim to be a new paradigm appears premature or over-inflated. The problems are both practical and conceptual. Implementation is slow and patchy. There is a paucity of high-quality evidence, nor is it evenly distributed. There are doubts about the extent to which bias can be excluded from research. Equally, the model has not adequately addressed the question of how evidence can be applied in practice or how evidence can be combined with practitioner experience and consumer perspectives. These problems have yet to be solved in medicine, and are probably even more difficult to tackle in other disciplines.

At the same time, however, it is too easy to dwell on the difficulties of evidence-based practice. The approach has responded to a significant problem of the gap between research and practice. The systematisation and dissemination of what is known makes obvious sense. Equally the movement has brought issues of research quality, transparency, accountability and consumer participation to the fore.

Significant questions remain. In particular, it remains unclear how the model can incorporate other knowledges or how evidence can be applied in real-world situations. One of the problems with evidence-based practice is that its rational scientific world-view constrains the answers it can supply. Evidence-based practice tends to fit solutions to problems into its own world-view, providing more and better information, further refinement of methodological criteria or incorporating consumer perspectives into an evidence-based practice framework. The result is that there are major outstanding issues that the rational scientific model is ill-equipped to handle, and would appear unlikely to resolve.

What is to be done? One of the problems of the debate around evidence-based practice is that both sides tend to get locked into a false binary of for or against, science or art, intervention or care, reason or emotion, quantitative or qualitative. Moving forward is likely to involve a strategy of both–and rather than either–or. The champions of evidence-based practice will need to recognise that there are other types of knowledge that cannot be ignored or fashioned in its own image. Equally the critics will need to recognise that, though imperfect, the knowledge provided by evidence-based practice can contribute to the development of practice.

Moving to a both–and position will require a broadening-out in the definition of evidence-based practice. The definitions of what constitutes evidence and the hierarchy of evidence require rethinking. Although evidence-based practice theoretically supports the matching of research designs to questions, in practice a cursory scan of evidence-based practice databases or journals indicates that it is only RCT data and meta-analysis that counts. The weaknesses of RCTs, particularly but not exclusively, in social interventions have been highlighted in this chapter. It is now time to consider how other research designs, including qualitative research, can be utilised fully. It is worth noting that a Cochrane qualitative methods group is in the process of formation (http://www.salford.ac.uk/ihr/cochrane/homepage.htm). It is vital, however, that qualitative and other research designs are accepted and valued on their own terms, rather than fitted awkwardly and inappropriately within an existing framework (see Chapter 6).

Research is an inherently political process. The tendency of the evidence-based practice movement has been to respond to this by trying to eliminate bias by technical means and further refinements of the review process to produce a somewhat false sense of certainty. Fuller attention to the issues and outcomes of concern to consumers will help. Just as important is a greater degree of reflexivity amongst researchers, reviewers and practitioners to think about what assumptions about the world are taken for granted and what questions and answers are not addressed or precluded by particular pieces of research or particular research designs.

In an uncertain world solutions which promise certainty have immense appeal. It is important that all evidence be treated with caution. The methodological rigour of evidence-based practice conveys a sense of certainty and authority. As we have seen, however, absolute certainty is rarely to be found. There are major areas where evidence is lacking, questions about the extent to which evidence can be trusted (meta-analysis), questions about the applicability of evidence in real-life cases, and concerns about the narrowness of evidence and narrowness of outcomes. In some areas certainty is more founded, whilst in other areas, beyond the biological, the search for certainty poses considerable dangers in inherently complex and uncertain worlds. Whilst evidence is potentially helpful it is important not be seduced into an unwarranted sense of security.

At the same time as the definition of evidence should be broadened, the scope or claims of evidence-based practice should be narrowed. At its birth evidence-based medicine was proclaimed as a new paradigm. Whatever the setting, evidence is just one aspect of decision-making, which has to be set alongside rather than appropriating other crucial components, especially professional expertise and consumer perspectives; it should also include economic considerations, ethics and the general policy framework. Sweeney's conclusion that evidence-based medicine is 'a necessary but not in itself a sufficient condition for the practice of good medicine in primary care' probably holds true for most disciplines (Sweeney 1996: 59).

The weight to be given to evidence and the centrality of evidence within practice is likely to vary by discipline. We have looked in this book at the potential evidence-based practice offers in a range of disciplines. Although the framework appears to be universally applicable, and has found passionate adherents in a range of disciplines, it does also appear that key aspects of the framework reflect its origins in acute medicine. In particular, it would seem that the population focus of RCT data, and the particular suitability of RCTs to pharmacological interventions and specialties, limits the scope of the model in areas where interventions are centred around webs of human relationships, and where much of the work is practical rather than technical. This is not to say that evidence and evidence-based practice has no place, but that its role may be less central and the conclusions drawn from evidence more uncertain. In practice, there are worrying signs that in some of the less powerful or autonomous disciplines, notably education and probation, evidence-based practice is in danger of becoming a means by which managers can force a particular and narrow definition of effective practice upon researchers and practitioners.

Probably the biggest challenge, however, is that of implementation. The evidence-based practice movement has had remarkable success in spreading its message widely in a short space of time. The development of practice has not followed a similar trajectory. The initial assumption that providing better and more digestible information would change practice has proved unrealistic. It is possible that the redefinition of evidence suggested here, and the redefinition of a new paradigm into an important component of a larger toolkit, might help to overcome some of the resistance to the approach, and to facilitate the informed consent that will be necessary for the incorporation of evidence into daily practice.

References

Bastian H. (1994) *The Power Of Sharing Knowledge: Consumer Participation in the Cochrane Collaboration*. Cochrane Consumer Collaboration.
http://som.flinders.edu.au/FUSA/COCHRANE/cochrane/powershr.htm

Black N. (1996) Why we need observational studies to evaluate the effectiveness of health care. *British Medical Journal*, **312**, 1215–18.

Carr-Hill R. (1995) Welcome? to the brave new world of evidence-based medicine. *Social Science and Medicine*, **41**, 1467–8.

Cochrane Collaboration Consumer Network (1998) *Cochrane Consumer Network Newsletter*, Issue 5. http://som.flinders.edu.au/FUSA/COCHRANE/newslett/cnnew5.htm

Coulter A., Entwistle V. & Gilbert D. (1999) Sharing decisions with patients: is the information good enough? *British Medical Journal*, **318**, 318–22.

Culpper L. & Gilbert T. (1999) Evidence and ethics. *Lancet*, **353**, 829–31.

Davis D., Thomson M., Oxman A. & Haynes R. (1995) Changing physician performance: a systematic review of continuing medical education strategies. *Journal of the American Medical Association*, **274**, 700–705.

Dawes M. (1996) On the need for evidence-based general and family practice. *Evidence-Based Medicine*, **1**, 68–9.

Donald A. (1998) *The Front-Line Evidence-Based Medicine Project*. Final Report. NHS Executive, North Thames Regional Office, London.

Dunning M., Abi-Aad G., Gilbert D., Gillam S. & Livett H. (1997) *Turning Evidence into Everyday Practice: an Interim Report from the PACE Programme*. The King's Fund Publishing, London.

Egger M., Davey-Smith G., Schneider M. & Minder C. (1997) Bias in meta-analysis detected by a simple, graphical test. *British Medical Journal*, **315**, 629–34.

Egger M., Davey-Smith G. (1997) Meta-analysis: potentials and promise. *British Medical Journal*, **315**, 1371–4.

Entwistle V.A., Renfrew M.J., Yearley S., Forrester J. & Lamont T. (1998a) Lay perspectives: advantages for health research. *British Medical Journal*, **316**, 463–6.

Entwistle V.A., Sheldon T.A., Sowden A. & Watt I.S. (1998b) Evidence-informed patient choice: practical issues of involving patients in decisions about health care technologies. *International Journal of Technology Assessment in Health Care*, **14**, 212–25.

Eve R., Golton I., Hodgkin P., Munro J. & Musson G. (1997) *Learning from Facts: Lessons from the Framework for Appropriate Care Throughout Sheffield (FACTS) Project*. ScHARR Occasional Paper no. 97/3. School of Health and Related Research, University of Sheffield, Sheffield.

Evidence-Based Medicine Working Group (1992) Evidence-based medicine: a new approach to teaching the practice of medicine. *Journal of the American Medical Association*, **268**, 2420–25.

Fisher B. (1998) How to utilise patients' views to influence service quality. *PACE Bulletin*, Special Issue, **June**. http://www.kingsfund.org.uk/PACE/spe98.htm

Glasziou P., Guyatt G.H., Dans A.L. *et al.* (1998) Applying the results of trials and systematic reviews to individual patients. *ACP Journal Club*, **129** (3), 15–16.

Godlee (1998) Applying research evidence to individual patients: evidence-based case reports will help [editorial]. *British Medical Journal*, **316**, 1621–2.

Grahame-Smith D. (1995) Evidence-based medicine: Socratic dissent. *British Medical Journal*, **310**, 1126–7.

Gray J.A.M. (1997) *Evidence-Based Healthcare: How to Make Health Policy and Management Decisions*. Churchill Livingstone, New York.

Greenhalgh T. (1997) *How to Read a Paper*. BMJ Publishing Group, London.

Greenhalgh T. & Hurwitz B. (1998) *Narrative-Based Medicine: Dialogue and Discourse in Clinical Practice*. BMJ Publishing Group, London.

Griffiths M. (1997) Must be applied critically [Letter]. *British Medical Journal*, **311**, 257.

Grol R. (1997) Beliefs and evidence in changing clinical practice. *British Medical Journal*, **31**, 418–21.

Haines B. & Haines A. (1998) Barriers and bridges to evidence-based clinical practice. *British Medical Journal*, **317**, 273–6.

Hampton J.R. (1997) Evidence-based medicine, practice variations and clinical freedom. *Journal of Evaluation in Clinical Practice*, **3**, 123–31.

Jacobson L., Edwards A., Granier S. & Bulter C. (1997) Evidence-based medicine and general practice. *British Journal of General Practice*, **47**, 449–52.

Jones G. & Sagar S. (1995) No guidance is provided for situations for which evidence is lacking [Letter]. *British Medical Journal*, **311**, 258.

Kerridge I., Lowe M. & Henry D. (1998) Ethics and evidence-based medicine. *British Medical Journal*, **316**, 1151–3.

Knottnerus J.A. & Dinant G.J. Medicine-based evidence: a prerequisite for evidence-based medicine. *British Medical Journal*, **315**, 1109–10.

Lancet (1995) Evidence-based medicine, in its place [Editorial]. *Lancet*, **346**, 785.

Macdonald G. (1996) Ice therapy: why we need randomised controlled trials. In P. Alderson, S. Brill, R. Fuller *et al.* (eds) *What Works? Effective Social Interventions in Child Welfare*. Barnardos, Barkingside.

Marteau T., Sowden A. & Armstrong D. (1998) Implementing research findings into practice: beyond the information deficit model. In A. Haines & A. Donald (eds) *Getting Research Findings into Practice*. BMJ Books, London.

Mayer J. & Timms N. (1970) *The Client Speaks*. Routledge and Kegan Paul, London.

McGuire J.B., Stein A. & Rosenberg W. (1997) Evidence-based medicine and child mental health services. *Children and Society*, **11**, 8996.

Meredith B. (1998) Informal survey on consumer involvement in the Cochrane Collaboration. *Cochrane Consumer Network Newsletter*, Issue **5**, http://som.flinders.edu.au/FUSA/COCHRANE/newslett/cnnew5.htm

Naylor D. (1997) Meta-analysis and the meta-epidemiology of clinical research: meta-analysis is an important contribution to research and practice but it's not a panancea [Editorial]. *British Medical Journal*, **315**, 617–19.

NHS Centre for Reviews and Dissemination (1994) *Implementing Clinical Guidelines*. Effective Health Care Bulletin, vol 1, no. 8. University of York, York.

NHS Centre for Reviews and Dissemination (1999) *Getting Evidence into Practice*. Effective Health Care Bulletin, vol 5, no. 1. University of York, York.

Norman G.R. & Shannon S.I. (1998) Effectiveness of instruction in critical appraisal (evidence-based medicine) skills: a critical appraisal. *Canadian Medical Association Journal*, **158**, 177–82.

Oxman A., Thomson M. & Davis D. (1995) No magic bullets: a systematic review of 102 trials of interventions to improve professional practice. *Canadian Medical Association Journal*, **153**, 1423–31.

Polychronis A., Miles A. & Bentley D.P. (1996a) Evidence-based medicine: Reference? Dogma? Neologism? New orthodoxy? *Journal of Evaluation in Clinical Practice*, **2**, 1–3.

Polychronis A., Miles A. & Bentley D.P. (1996b) The protagonists of EBM: arrogant, seductive and controversial. *Journal of Evaluation in Clinical Practice*, **2**, 9–12.

Rosenberg W. & Donald A. (1995a) Authors' reply. *British Medical Journal*, **311**, 259.

Rosenberg W. & Donald A. (1995b) Evidence-based medicine: an approach to clinical problem solving. *British Medical Journal*, **310**, 1122–6.

Sackett D. & Haynes R. (1995) On the need for evidence-based medicine. *Evidence-Based Medicine*, **1**, 5.

Sackett D.L., Rosenberg W.M., Gray J.A., Haynes R.B. & Richardson W.S. (1996) Evidence-based medicine: what it is and what it isn't [Editorial]. *British Medical Journal*, **312**, 71–2.

Shahar E. (1997) A Popperian perspective on the term 'evidence-based medicine'. *Journal of Evaluation in Clinical Practice*, **3**, 109–16.

Sheldon T., Guyatt G. & Haines A. (1998) When to act on the evidence. *British Medical Journal*, **317**, 139–42.

Smith G. & Cantley C. (1985) *Assessing Health Care*. Open University Press, Buckingham.

Smith B. & Taylor R. (1996) Medicine: a healing or a dying art? *British Journal of General Practice*, **46**, 249–51.

Sullivan F. & MacNaughton R. (1996) Evidence in consultations: interpreted and individualised. *Lancet*, **348**, 941–3.

Sweeney K. (1996) Evidence and uncertainty. In M. Marinker (ed.) *Sense and Sensibility in Health Care*. BMJ Publishing Group, London.

Tannenbaum S. (1993) What physicians know. *New England Journal of Medicine*, **329**, 1268–71.

Taubes G. (1996) Looking for the evidence in medicine. *Science*, **272**, 22–4.

Thoburn J., Lewis A. & Shemmings D. (1995) *Paternalism or Partnership: Family Involvement in the Child Protection Process*. HMSO, London.

Wise J. (1997) Health authority stops buying homeopathy. *British Medical Journal*, **314**, 1574.

Index